D0207011

TRIUMPH OVER HEPATITIS C

PART 1:

How American doctor's deal with Hepatitis C.
The Perspective of one patient determined to be Hepatitis C Free.

PART 2:

The Remedy:
The Alternative Medicine Solution that saved my life.

LLOYD WRIGHT

PUBLISHED BY:
LLOYD WRIGHT
P. O. Box 6347
Malibu, CA 90264
877-676-1615
LLOYDHEPCFREE@MSN.COM

1ST Printing June 1999
7th Printing September 2000
Revised Edition

DISCLAIMER

It is not our intention or purpose to replace the service of a physician, nor is it our purpose to guarantee any medical or nutritional preparation or the effectiveness thereof. The information in this book is not presented with the intention of diagnosing or prescribing. It is intended to help those who wish to cooperate with their physician in a mutual desire to build and maintain health. We believe that in the event someone uses this information without his or her doctor's approval, doing this for him or herself, he or she is only exercising their constitutional right to pursue happiness. Therefore, the author, editors and publisher assume no responsibility.

All rights reserved. No part of this book may be reproduced by any means or in any from, except brief quotes for literary reviews, without permission from the publisher.

COPYWRITE LLOYD WRIGHT 1999
TRIUMPH OVER HEPATITIS C
AN ALTERNATIVE MEDICINE SOLUTION

ISBN 0-9676404-1-5

Forward

By Dr. John Finnegan, N.D.*

The health of the world population is deteriorating at an accelerating rate due to humankind's pervasive pollution of their environment, a depletion of nutrients in the soils and food, and an imbalance in our way of living. Yet in the midst of this darkness of our own creation there is the dawning light of a special knowledge of herbs and nutrients. These herbs and nutrients can give protection and healing to those who strive to live consciously, and who are open to appreciate God's creations in nature.

Mr. Lloyd Wright has written an account of his journey from infection with Hepatitis C through his becoming Hepatitis C free. He is one who went to the extreme to conquer his life-threatening ailment. He diligently practiced all of the pertinent knowledge he obtained. Regardless of the peril necessary to acquire funds, Mr. Wright reached beyond the medical establishment of the 20th century to obtain the knowledge necessary to continue living.

The FDA's only approved drug for Hepatitis C is interferon. The use of this isolated, single action drug creates imbalances in the body's digestive and immune systems as well as interference with brain function, triggering a domino effect of dysfunction and deterioration throughout the entire body. Keep in mind, there is nothing more powerful or holistically designed than our body's own system for growth, health, defense and healing.

While the medical professional's drugs are becoming less effective and more harmful, it is evident that there is a tremendous need for health practitioners to look to holism and alternative methods that are effective against disease while at the same time strengthening the immune system and supporting the body's overall health.

Many people, including medical practitioners, feel that herbs are "good for" minor things, but don't have the capacity to help the body fight serious diseases. In fact, there are many herbal therapies that have profound effects on curing even the most serious disease. Mr. Wright provides a valuable service by identifying these in his book.

People and doctors rely on pharmaceuticals because this is what they know. Yet it has been reported by the American Medical Association ('98) that even when taken properly, prescription medicines account for 100,000 deaths each year and a million hospitalizations. We accept these pharmaceuticals as our "health care" treatments even though they can cause serious imbalances and harmful side effects that impact our quality of health and life

Traditional medicine certainly has its place as a crisis intervention when the body is traumatically hurt or is seriously failing. However, nutritional and herbal therapies should certainly be considered and tried before resorting to invasive and costly medicines and treatments.

A lack of awareness and education, in addition to misinformation by both the pharmaceutical and the natural products industries, as well as poorly processed natural products have kept most of us in the dark about the proper use and possibilities for effective herbal remedies.

Mr. Wright's long and costly journey through the dark halls of traditional medicine led him to discover and try these herbal and alternative remedies. Had he not, he would be dead today.

Dr. John Finnegan, N.D.

*John Finnegan, N.D. is a Doctor of Naturopathic Medicine, researcher, and author of 10 books presenting his work in the holistic health sciences. His previous works, "The Facts about Fats" and "Recovery From Addiction" have received widespread professional recognition.

Introduction

Hepatitis C is a life-threatening virus. Doctors are treating hepatitis C as if this were the *DARK AGES*. They treat Hep. C patients with Interferon, even though this "therapy" and all its combinations have proven to be a complete failure. Rather than recognizing the value of natural therapies, they recommend to thousands of patients to simply wait for a liver transplant. Many die waiting. Many more die from other complications from hepatitis C, which a liver transplant cannot help.

Fortunately, in the 21st century man has re-discovered time proven natural healing. We, as a culture, are becoming more aware of the fact that we can support our immune systems. We can boost our immune systems to help it achieve what it does best ...heal.

I believe that through knowledge and persistence we can achieve optimum health. Unfortunately it can take time, money and sacrifice to acquire the necessary supplements, but you can't wait! The following letter is being published to make this point. Don't waste your time worrying about money. Instead, use your time to make more time. Do something. Read on.

May 25, 2000

Hello Lloyd,

Regarding my telephone conversations with you in the recent days-I can't begin to tell you how much your kindness and compassion meant to me. Your sharing of information as to what I could do to possibly help my husband while he was in the hospital was sincerely appreciated. It's nice to know that there are amongst the human population pockets of truly good, kind and selfless individuals striving to help others without the obvious ulterior motives (and we know what those are). You are an angel!

My husband passed away last Wednesday, on May 17th. During the last week of his life my frantic research led me to four different methods of helping his condition, one of which was yours, and all the people involved with these methods were the kindest of individuals. I felt blessed having made their acquaintance. But unfortunately it was too little – too late. My husband lingered in the hospital for four weeks and so did I. The nurses managed to scrape up a cot for me and as I slept there each night by his bed, time became irrelevant.

My daughter, who is 21, came up with the idea of having an alternative funeral service for him, which I wholeheartedly supported. I've been a "truth-seeker" and pursuing the spiritual path for 20 years now and my daughter Jamie is following a similar course (though she's far wiser at her age than I ever was – I find many of the young are further ahead in wisdom than many adults ever were at their age). And so we put together a beautiful service, which we referred to not as a funeral but a "rebirth celebration."

This became so appropriate since my husband had given myself, and my children, the most treasured of all gifts. (You must understand here that he was a man of few words, incredibly strong, never complained when he felt pain, and a businessman to boot/ type A personality. The only time he verbally rattled on was when it involved speaking about his business, which was the audio/visual business. And as for spirituality and such as seeing through the "veil of illusion" (I remembered you liked that expression) it was another world for him...But when he went into his first coma on "Good Friday" we, my daughter and I, prayed like hell hoping to bring him back to consciousness and healing. Well, Easter Sunday he regained his consciousness. The following day Jamie had asked her father very casually what he had experienced during his coma. He looked into her eyes, pulled the covers up around his neck and said very seriously, "Jamie I know this might sound crazy but it's true what they say. In a flash I found myself in the most beautiful magical world you could ever imagine. I was dancing and playing and singing. I have never felt so free and happy in all my life. It was soooo beautiful." She then asked if he had seen a white light and he replied, "Oh yes the white light was there, but it was unlike any white light you could ever imagine in this physical world." She then asked if he had a choice to come back and he said, "Yes, I did have a choice but I was enjoying myself so much that I really didn't want to come back. But eventually everything started to fade and here I am." Apparently he confided in her that he had many such experiences but he could only just remember the one to tell her at that time. This was the gift he gave us, to let us know that his passing didn't mean him fading off into some oblivion or deep, dark hole. It was the absolute knowing that he has passed on to some wonderfully, happy, magical world; a world he expressed to Jamie as being "better than Disney world." This truly comforts us during terrible times of missing him. No amount of money could put a price on this.

The guests were informed not to come in black, but lighter colors and we incorporated nature into the service to emphasize the cycle of rebirth. We had wonderful feedback from all who attended that it was the most beautiful "funeral" they had ever attended. It was truly and in every aspect a celebration of who he was and a celebration of life, which is something he always wished to do, but which the Hepatitis C deprived him of.

But just the same, with him gone now I feel as if I've been jettisoned into the "Twilight Zone", one moment they're here and the next they're gone forever.

Lloyd, thank you so much for your book and all of the photocopies! I received them in the mail yesterday and have begun to read the book. Fabulous!!! I can feel your heart and soul in it!!!! What a nightmare you experienced and it makes me understand so much more of what excruciating hell my husband experienced all those years without ever letting me know the full truth of what was happening to him. (I will explain this at a further date; his determination to protect his wife and children became a destructive, misinformed obsession).

Understanding what torture you experienced made me understand why in those days before he entered the hospital it was as if I were looking into the eyes of a drowning man. He was literally drowning in his own bodily fluids. The lymphatic fluids that had been accumulating in his body over the last several years had been mistaken for body fat. His legs became so water logged that he could barely walk and his penis disappeared into his pubic area somewhere. The poor man was at his wits end wondering why his thighs and legs kept ballooning. He had constant abscesses between his thighs that would break open and bleed. His problems were numerous. It was hell for me because subconsciously I knew he was a dying man (looking into his eyes was torture) and I couldn't figure out what was wrong. But I believe he was quite confused himself in spite of the fact that he knew he had Hepatitis C. He had a list of more than a dozen doctors he'd been seeing. Goodness knows what they told him. It's all guesswork for me now. But suffer, did he ever!

I intend at some point to get in touch with you again because I would like to help expose your book to Hepatitis C patients here in Toronto. So when my life and finances are in order, I will order several copies for those looking for the help you offer. I will mention your name whenever I can, for you deserve it! I'll need time to come to terms with this new direction in my life now, so when I'm back on top of things I'll connect again.

Thanks for being the champion you are! We need brave men like you, there are far too few in the world today!

Yours truly,
Debra Capranos

Acknowledgments

While it has been almost six years since I began documenting the ballistic treachery that has plagued my life since my diagnosis of Hepatitis C to my recovery, I have strived to shape a piece of written material that could help other people faced with this seemly impossible mission to know that Hep. C can be overcome!

I stood alone in a world of non-believing Medical Doctors.

In this Revised Edition I honor my editor, Aunika Stratton. She has spent many hours correcting my many spelling and grammatical errors and put up with my relentless behavior. Her contribution has made this revised edition easier to understand, and provides the reader with many new items that were the most frequently asked questions from previous readers.

My special thanks go out to Irwin Zucker for bringing my quest to millions of Americans through Radio and T.V. programs.

A huge thanks to Shannon Rice for the grueling hours she spent formatting this book and for making my website a tremendous success.

Thanks to the special people who practiced my Remedy and have called, E-mailed and written expressing gratitude and endless thanks for their normal liver panels and return to normal life!

My thanks to my readers, who can overlook the fact that I am not a doctor, or a literary genius, just a person who found an answer.

Special thanks to Dr. Yeast de Villars, Dr. Miller, Dr. Nichols, Dr. John Finnegan, Dr. Ed Wagner and Dr. Debar Banker.

I would like to thank Dr. Roy for telling me to THINK. He wrote it on a paper, circled it and it is still on my refrigerator today. Dr. Roy's suggestions have transformed my life.

This book is dedicated to
Pattie, for reasons that need
not be explained here, to
the men and women of
Fire Station 56 and to
Bob Dylan
for *Political World.*

TRIUMPH

OVER

HEPATITIS

C

AN ALTERNATIVE MEDICINE SOLUTION

REVISED EDITION

Table of Contents

Part I

Exposing the Ignorance and Arrogance of the Medical Industry

Chapter 1	1979-1980	25
Chapter 2	1983-1991	27
Chapter 3	1993	35
Chapter 4	1995	39
Chapter 5	On A Quest	45
Chapter 6	1996	51
Chapter 7	Hepatitis C Researcher	55
Chapter 8	Media Hype	63
Chapter 9	PATS Report	67
Chapter 10	The Letter	73
Chapter 11	Dark Ages	89

Part II
The Remedy

Chapter 12 Milk Thistle **101**

Chapter 13 Thymus **105**

Chapter 14 Bovine Liver **109**

Chapter 15 Reishi Mushrooms **125**

Chapter 16 Alpha-Lipoic Acid (ALA) **129**

Chapter 17 Licorice Root **133**

Chapter 18 Dandelion Root **137**

Chapter 19 Cats Claws **139**

Chapter 20 Aloe Vera **143**

Chapter 21 Vitamin C **165**

Chapter 22 Alfalfa **171**

Chapter 23 NADH **173**

Chapter 24 Albumin **175**

Chapter 25 Foods to Help You be Hepatitis C Free 181

Chapter 26 Things to Avoid 187

Summary 197

Testimonials 199

References 215

Appendices

Appendix A 223
The liver in Health and Disease

Appendix B 245
Hepastat Ingredients
Hepata Trope Ingredients

Appendix C 257
Study results with Thymosin

Appendix D 261
Alfalfa Leaf Ingredients

Addendums

Addendum 1 263
Blood Swap Helps Severe MS

Addendum 2 265
A Conflict of Interest

Part I

Ignorance and Arrogance of the Medical Industry

Chapter One

1979-1980

During the late summer of 1979, September 9th to be exact, I fell through the gates of Hell while operating my newly purchased John Deere tractor.

The "yellow monster" suffered catastrophic mechanical failure: the hydraulic reverse system had failed, summoning Lucifer himself.

Backwards it thundered, flipping over and launching me behind it as it went thrashing through the bushes, careening down a thousand-foot cliff.

I was crushed as the sixteen thousand pound piece of American junk rolled over me on a very steep, remote site in the Santa Monica Mountains.

There were no people or houses within miles. Blood gushed from my pants as if I were wading in it. My vision went black and white, or probably more gray. I felt very peaceful, and lay down to die.

To my surprise, a lone horseback rider at a great distance had seen this happen. He had a small CB radio and made a call. Within several minutes a medivac helicopter landed. With much effort they carted me up the hill on a stretcher. All I remembered about what happened was that my guard dog, Jerome, leaped in the helicopter on top of my body and then began attacking my rescuers.

I woke up in Los Robles hospital. I'm told it was the only hospital at the time in the Western Hemisphere with two hyperberic chambers. This was experimental medicine to prevent crushed tissue from dying.

The surgeon on duty said my leg was broken in at least six different places, and my massive crush injury probably would result in kidney failure and death.

Over the next thirty days, I underwent nine major surgeries to reattach my leg. I received four blood transfusions and, unknown at the time, a lethal dose of Hepatitis C.

Chapter Two

1983-1991

In 1983, my doctors took away my pain medication, percodan. They said my liver was inflamed. I was in extreme pain, and was told that I was going to have to learn to live with it. This news was a little hard for me to handle. I build houses and was creating a forty-acre avocado ranch. The doctors wouldn't give me any more drugs. Those doctors should be shot and wounded, left to flounder until death. Perhaps then they would understand the need for drugs in our sick 90's culture.

They prescribed a mood elevator called Desyrel (Trazodone) HCI. In a few months, I was paranoid about going to the local market. I found myself in bed with a large woman and her daughter.

Seven years passed. My physician told me my liver count was a little high, but there was no cause for worry. In 1991 I was diagnosed with malignant testicular lymphoma, cancer. Oh joy, they were going to castrate me.

During radiation therapy, the Oncologist told me my liver count was so high that I must be a serious alcoholic. I denied the charge. After therapy, he continued to monitor my liver count. At one point he said it was so high that I must be an intravenous drug user.

I informed him that I had never stuck a needle in my body, and my alcohol intake was negligible. After much debate, the Oncologist tested me for Hepatitis C. It was July 7, 1991. The first type of Hepatitis C test was an inaccurate test. My result was negative. In September of that same year, the Hepatitis C test was perfected; however, no one retested me!

Well now, here I was, my body crushed and nearly castrated. If that's not bad enough, my insurance company canceled my policy, and I didn't have any family to help me; they all died from cancer, except my father. I truly love him, but he didn't make grants.

After two months of 180 rads of radiation a day, I couldn't function. I was supposed to eat well, but I didn't have any money. Ever pay cash to get neutered and radiated? Well, I got a real deal because I paid cash for the initial clipping.

I met a decent, honest doctor, and he did it in an outpatient facility for twelve hundred dollars cash.

Right before they "put me under", the doc handed me a form giving him the right to cut whatever cancer he found. That meant I could wake up without "JR". Well, that's a wonderful way to "go under".

I was given morphine, my drug of choice, for signing away my "masculinity" for a plastic tube.

They prepared me for a shave. The lady who prepared me could have shaved a t-rex. Talk about a monster, in fact she could have used a shave her self.

Thankfully I only saw her for a few moments. Actually I wish I knew her, best shave I've ever had.

Twelve hours later I woke up on a bed. There I was, in the middle of this sea of recovering patients, a row of beds in each direction for as far as I could see.

My first mission, reach down and feel, hopefully, something that was there before. Thank God, "JR" was still there. The right testicle didn't make it, but the left did.

The next crisis, I had to urinate at least half a cup before they would let me out of this God forsaken body part removal facility. Hours, I'd say six, and I just could not do it. Finally, I faked it with two drops of urine and half a glass of water. "JR" has functioned great ever since, and in fact, maybe better.

They gave me a few weeks to recover, a bottle of percodan, and added no alcohol or sex for six weeks. Upon arriving home, my female sex partner was waiting. They must have used steel stitches because that "she creature" did everything in her power to break them loose.

I mean, imagine a bottle of percodan, a case of Dom Perignom, and a wild, crazy Latino. "JR" went for days.

The rads really took a toll on me though. I couldn't do anything except drive to and from the hospital, five days a week. It took one hour to get there, one hour to get back and an eternity while I "got zapped".

During this time there was much debate between my Oncologist and me. First, about what he supposed to be my serious alcohol problem. I mean he thought I was a "sterno user". Then he suspected me of being an intravenous drug user, all because my liver tests were outrageous. I liked to party, but I didn't sit around drinking all day, and I never shot drugs.

This man, a Radiation Oncologist, was a rocket scientist before becoming a doctor. Back in the 70's he worked on the space shuttle. One day he decided he wanted to "nuke" people. He spent some time in New Mexico, and bingo, he's an Oncologist.

He knew nothing about blood transfusions or Hepatitis. Apparently he didn't even know that the first Hepatitis C tests performed were as accurate as Sitting Bull shooting an arrow at the moon.

The Hepatitis C test wasn't perfected until September 1991, but did anyone ever think of retesting me? No! Did any future doctor ever realize that my negative test result was one of the unreliable ones? Of all the doctors I saw, not one even knew anything about this until I saw a state appointed psychiatrist/neurologist, who was working on the Gulf War Syndrome.

Four years after the first test I saw this doctor when I was being reviewed for the second time for disability. The state thought I was crazy because, under the topic of sports I practiced daily, I wrote masturbation.

This brings me to my second encounter with the Federal government. Broke and hungry, I figured I had paid social security all my life, more than most because I was self-employed. I've paid lots of property tax, and I went to the welfare office for my zip code, right by the Federal building in LA.

I parked and walked to the door. Two large "uniformed officers" were on each side of a metal detector. I was frisked and felt up; the only white boy there and I think the "officers" really enjoyed this.

I got the forms, filled them out, and sat waiting for my name to be called.

A young black man sitting next to me began to laugh uncontrollably. After he slowed down he sneaked a can of "Bud" out of his coat pocket and took a sip. So much for the metal detector!

He said, "What's wrong with you white boy? You got shrimp for brains? You can't have an address and get nothing." Then he cracked up again. "White boy, you got shrimp for brains. You got to get another form. You can't have a bank account and get something from these fools. White boy, you got to get a new form. I'll help you. You got to lie. You got to lie or you get nothing. They don't give a rat's ass about your gonads. You got to tell them you got no home, no brains, no nothing and they got to believe you is crazy."

Well, I decided not to lie; and yes, he who lied got. I got nothing. So much for Social Security. I thought the Federal government should shove off and fry in hell, at least as far as proclaiming that there was medical help available for any one who needed it.

The Federal government didn't help me in this crisis. I didn't make any money during this time, and I was suffering badly. The silent killer, Hepatitis C, was working on me and no one knew it. The government sent me to a doctor in Los Angeles for screening for Supplemental Security Income (SSI); it was late 1991.

He was a pulmonary doctor. I was sent there because of my liver and testicular cancer! I was very puzzled as to why they sent me to a "lung" doctor for my liver and testicular cancer.

He examined me. His advice; stop taking vitamins A, C, D, E, and K; and your liver count will fall.

Was this why I paid taxes? Was this why SSI was developed?

Today, please go die somewhere and leave us alone. This doctor had all my records. He knew about blood transfusions, and he knew about Hepatitis C, didn't he? Maybe he didn't?

I'm a contractor, and I know my trade. When I paint the outside of a house, I don't use watercolors.

My personal belief is that these fools who practice medicine should be paid less than I am because I'm not practicing. I know my profession.

Don't get me wrong, I admire a good mechanic, which is all a good doctor can be. For the most part, fixing body parts is the only thing they really learn how to do. They can't cure viruses e.g. the common cold.

I was dying from a yet unknown cause, and I was told to stop consuming vitamins!

Refused by Medi-Cal. No program available for single white males between 21-65 existed.

Chapter Three

1993

For two years I felt I never recovered from radiation therapy. I had 180 rads a day for two months over most of my lymph system, and I never felt well again.

In 1993, I was building a house, my own house. In the past, when I built a house, especially my own house, I loved it. I would work twelve hours a day and on weekends as well. Now, I could not make it through the day. I was tired and I felt sick. I complained, mostly to my primary physician, that I could no longer drink any alcohol at all because it made me sick.

He responded, "That's good. The stuff is bad for you anyway."

After three years of being tired and more tired, breaking fingernails, hair falling out, becoming dizzy and having sweats at night, to the point of my entire bed being soaked; the doctor told me I probably just needed a rest.

I went to a Gastroenterologist, Dr. D. I ended up there because my dentist gave me an antibiotic that caused bleeding lesions in my colon. All my blood ended up in the toilet. He inserted a giant silver prod into my anal canal, devastating my posterior rectum for at least a year, and he never even apologized. I was instantly considered a drug addict for even asking for any pain medication. I noticed several large books about the liver on his shelves, so I mentioned my high liver panel numbers from years earlier.

After extensive diagnoses, he decided that I had too much iron in my liver, and I began having weekly phlebotomies. I went to a blood bank once a week and had my blood sucked out. It was supposed to be discarded as toxic waste.

One fine day, someone screwed up and placed my blood with the donation blood, and it was randomly tested.

Two months later, the blood bank sent me a letter stating I could no longer donate blood because I had Hepatitis C. What a surprise!

The first thing I did was to call the blood bank and ask for someone who could answer some questions for me. I was transferred to a technician, who said he knew quite a bit about Hepatitis C. He graciously explained that I could expect to die from Hepatitis C or hepatocellular carcinoma, a complication of Hepatitis C. He said there was no cure, and I would suffer a slow death from internal bleeding and flu-like symptoms. It would be a long, slow demise, regardless of the path the disease took.

That was really exciting news!

Over-the-phone diagnoses often inspire me. It led me to believe that there were these small minded fools, presiding in offices all over the country just waiting to deliver some devastating news to the first person they can. It's like a collection agency that proclaims, you're going to live under a bridge when they're through with you, for being a day late on your credit card payments.

I took my test results to two doctors; first, my general practitioner. I asked him what was it, and what should I do about it? He said, "I don't know. Let me look into it, and I'll get back to you."

Then I went back to Dr. D whom I had seen before, with my test results and asked him the same questions. I received the same answer, but he did get back to me right away.

He advised me that since I had no insurance I should go directly to the county hospital. I assured him that was not an option. I was not about to let some county employee prolong my suffering or hasten my demise.

He then explained to me about Interferon alfa-2B recombinant, the only Federal Drug Administration (FDA) approved medication for Hepatitis C. He said it had some side effects, but nothing serious, and it had a cure rate of eighty percent. (Refer to Appendix A for information on Interferon).

Every other day I was to inject three million units of this medication in a different place in my body. I went to the pharmacy and purchased a two-week supply, six vials for $692.00.

In just one week, I was transformed into a monster. My head was exploding. My brain was landing on anyone who was nearby. I'd cry and different parts of my body would sweat. My head would be completely soaked, while my penis had icicles on it. I'd stay in bed for days. I could not function, and God help anyone who called on the phone.

I reported my intolerance to the doctor; he cut my dose in half.

Meanwhile, in an attempt to conserve the outflow of my dwindling supply of cash, I applied for a program supported by the drug manufacturer and the government, called Commitment To Care. This program was designed to help people without insurance who were in need of this wonder drug. I received a really nice letter of rejection, indicating that anyone with a Malibu address did not qualify.

Chapter Four

1995

Dr. D. ordered a liver biopsy.

The doctor that performed the test told me that I wouldn't even know it happened. He then injected a needle about two feet long and about the diameter of an ink pen, into my liver without any drugs. I swore that man would die and burn in hell. It was like being shot by the flaming arrow of a wild Indian. Later, I was told I wasn't given any pain medication because I was a cash patient.

As I lay there dying, the young and inexperienced doctor, I'll call "Pocahontas", decided to give me a percodan.

I want to know what these fools learn in school? Do they just stick needles in cadavers all day? Jesus Christ, this slime ball injected something the size of a primitive arrow into my side, guided it into my liver and didn't give me any medication to dull the pain. Was one painkiller going to turn me into a heroin addict? Was the bastard afraid the Drug Enforcement Agency (DEA) was going to jail him for intoxicating a patient? Perhaps it's just my karma? I'm supposed to suffer?

I can't, for one minute, understand what goes on in the heads of those mechanics, i.e. doctors, who think of themselves as little "gods".

Why did the government pay drug companies to develop the drugs, so only the drug dealers could profit or so that insurance companies could rake in hundreds of dollars per pill?

I think these small-minded "gods" should be required to be patients themselves and in class, have their classmates stick one of those "arrows" in their sides without drugs. Let them beg for death. Actually, considering their mentality, they may just become supporters of Dr. Kevorkian rather than drug conscious.

The most important part to understand is that cash patients are treated differently than insurance and welfare patients. Welfare patients are probably given some generic non-narcotic drug such as vicoden; unless it is a woman with a child, in that case she will probably get morphine and childcare.

The insurance patients never know anything happened to them, get an overnight stay in a plush suite, along with several rides up and down the hall in a wheelchair.

If the cash patient had a voice (and until now they haven't), this would not be the case. They don't want us to have one either. After all, doctors are human, even though they don't think so. I think some doctors have a need, a deep-seated desire to hurt someone, and they can do it to the cash patient and get away with it.

After arranging a ride home with my girlfriend Patty, she arrived at the hospital. Dr "Pocahontas" told her, "You have to stay with him for twenty-four hours because he could bleed to death. You cannot leave him. If he changes in any way, you must call and bring him here right away."

Patty took me home, and I fell asleep. I woke up a little while later, and she was gone. I was alone without a car. The nearest neighbor was a mile away. I started to walk to the nearest neighbor because I figured that was where she was. I'm pissed! I didn't knock; I just walked right in, ready to kill. After all, I've got America's best answer to Hepatitis C in my blood: Interferon alfa-2b recombinant.

Sure enough, there she was. She was "snorting" cocaine, a joint in one hand and a mug of some good hard liquor in the other. She was sitting there, deciding which of the several young males surrounding her would be her next victim. I could see it in her eyes.

Driven by the wonder drug, I was vicious. My look nearly killed her and a few innocent bystanders. I swear there are a few unfortunate people out there who probably had heart attacks and strokes that were induced by me while I was under the influence of Interferon.

During the entire year of 1995, I actually completed two weeks of full doses and ten weeks of half doses.

I also destroyed everyone I knew. I called my girlfriend's husband and told him I was having sex with his wife. I informed him that I had been having sex with her since their wedding day, when he passed out, and she went looking for someone to abuse.

Interferon destroyed my brain. My left knee felt like it had a blowtorch on it for months. I almost crashed my truck on several occasions. I got sicker and sicker until I swear I was almost dead. Yes, I'm convinced I was within hours of death.

Early in 1983, I was working at Carol Merril's restaurant, the Whale Watch. I could barely walk. As soon as she saw me she insisted on taking me to see Dr. Ed Wagner, a Chiropractor and healer. He practiced in his own home, just around the corner from The Whale Watch.

For four years I could not stand up and walk like a normal person. I was taking numerous and different medications for this problem. Attempting to avoid surgery, I went to Dr. Wagner, and he prescribed chiropractic manipulations and an extensive diet.

After about three weeks of his treatment, I was walking just fine. Now, after sixteen years I rarely have back pain, something eleven surgeons told me could be relieved only by surgery.

Nearly every time over the last sixteen years when I left Dr Wagner's office, I felt that something happened that I didn't understand. So many times I walked down his driveway, wondering what went on in there that caused me to feel so good?

When your spine is adjusted properly, your entire outlook, mood, attitude and feelings change for the better. You feel good! I believe his type of treatment was beneficial to my triumph over Hepatitis C.

I bought a computer and spent hours on the Internet searching for information about Hepatitis C. It was astounding to discover how much was being done around the world for Hepatitis C, with great results, but not in the U.S.

I had a neighbor, Jon Chann, who for months tried to convince me that I should see a Dr. John Finnegan, N.D. (Naturopathic Medicine). Finally I agreed. At the same time I made an appointment with a Hepatologist at Cedar Sinai Medical Center.

Chapter Five

On A Quest

About seventy-five miles north of Los Angeles, Patty had a burger fit. Malicious ball-busting female, I should have left her at home. She had no less than fifteen burger fits between Los Angeles and San Jose. Anywhere there was a Burger King or an In & Out Burger, this woman would threaten to orgasm, if I stopped.

The people out there on Highway 5 are different. Their goals are from a 1950's movie, Godzilla. These people hadn't been to college. They had spent their lives aspiring to work pumping gas at the local truck stop. They'd reached their goal, and it can be dangerous dealing with a person who has reached their goal, especially when they are half your age.

Between burgers, Patty had a gallon of milk mixed with two quarts of Kahlua, disguised in an ice chest. That woman can suck down more liquor than any man I've ever known or heard of. Patty's gone now, dead I think. Probably though, she's living somewhere like Laguna Beach, just millimeters from being institutionalized.

Patty was never any fun on a road trip. She believed she could only fly first class or ride in a limo. This trip, five hundred miles in a Toyota truck, was the low point of her miserable existence. However, we had a common destination. She was the bridesmaid at Kathy and Chris' wedding in Saratoga, September 7, 1996 while I was hunting for the west coast distributor of live cell Thymus, the main ingredient necessary to conquer Hepatitis C. San Mateo was my destination. My quest: to convince the highest person in that company that I had to have Thymus to survive.

I am a carpenter and could not afford to pay quadruple inflated prices for it. After all, we are talking about a very expensive cut of beef. This is not something regulated by the FDA.

We arrived in San Jose. Don't ever go there. The people there were either from hell or were, I'm sure, going there. We checked in. Patty was not happy. No room service and no elevator, it was very primitive. She woke up, called the nearest liquor store, ordered everything that would fit on my credit card and had it delivered. I went to sleep.

It was six a.m., September 5, 1996. I knew Ms. Patty wouldn't be awake until four p.m. so I went to San Mateo. Driving was so much easier when I didn't have a big, drunken lizard sharing the front and only seat. I arrived. I had called ahead and made an appointment with a Mr. Q. He told me he was really sorry, but he had a contract to distribute this product only to health care practitioners.

I had anticipated his response and had a very real and appreciative saga, which I delivered to him. I attempted to appeal to his human characteristics. He didn't have any. I got what I expected. Now it was back to hell or at least to the gathering area for those headed there.

I dared not awaken the drunken lizard, for admiration of life was something still securely attached to my being. Slowly though, she awoke and floundered around for a long while. She decided that she deserved a dinner in a fine French Bistro.

When it came to spending someone else's money, she was very professional. She collected herself, examined the yellow pages and called her friends in the wedding party. Her main objective was not to greet or say hello, but to locate the most expensive, elegant French restaurant within a sixty-mile radius. She was successful. She got directions, painted on make up and we were off. I was dying. I could feel that there were maybe only a few hours of this life left. I had felt this way often over about two years. Saratoga, with its quaint tree-lined streets, was a lovely place to die. I parked my truck, my lovely reliable Toyota truck. It always started and ran. If America made cars more like it, we'd still own Hawaii.

The following had to be told to me by Patty because I do not remember it.

She said that I could not sit in the chair. I kept sliding down and passing out, with my eyes open. I ordered a half bottle of non-alcoholic wine. She told me that I could not remember anything. I had not had any drugs or alcohol for who knew how long. I did remember the outside of the building, the streets and the trees. I also remembered the peace. The nearness of death, and the peace it promised. I felt very sick almost all the time.

The only reason I could put up with that drunken lizard was because I was too sick to dump her, which was good for her.

I didn't remember the food. She said it was good. We walked down the street while she smoked several cigarettes before the ride home, as there was no smoking in my truck. I was sick, and couldn't understand why she was trying to get sick. This woman smoked every conscious moment and consumed any and all available alcohol or drugs. She generally felt miserable, at least twenty-six days a month. All I was searching for was life. It was times such as these that I truly was ashamed that I haven't spent more time attempting to be a doctor of anything, at least perhaps my vocabulary would be such that I could express my true feelings more appropriately.

September 6th was the first and only time I had been instructed by Patty to awaken her before dark. We were off to brunch. The wedding party had invited about thirty-five people for brunch. It was back to Saratoga. What a wonderful group of people. It's very rare to meet so many wonderful people, all in one room.

The brunch was very casual, with plenty of champagne and any thing you wanted on the menu you could have with no restrictions. This was truly a celebration. Even though I was practically comatose, I remembered the grace, generosity, and celebration to which these people were dedicated. I've only read about such an event.

That evening in Saratoga, we were at the finest restaurant in town, and could have all the food we ever wanted. The father of the bride was a very happy man. Truly he was a great man by anointing his daughter and soon-to-be, son-in-law and all their friends with such a great event. There was an extraordinary feeling of well-being and friendship in the air. This friendliness and appreciation was felt by all.

I was very embarrassed about people wondering what was wrong with me. Yet, as sick as I was, I remembered that this event was as good, I'm sure, as going to heaven would be.

The next morning we were off to some former Senator's house for the final celebration. It was very nice, except that Ms. Patty, while dressing, had a romp with her male counterpart in the ladies' bathroom. Not what one would ponder from a traveling partner, during what were most certainly his final days.

Dedication was something with which the newly weds were adorned. Ms. Patty lacked it, in fact swore it would make her vomit.

There was another dinner after the wedding, in a remote place on a large creek. It was a great setting. Patty was off somewhere else. People had now seen me enough and had been introduced to me. They began to ask, "What is wrong with you?" I told them I had a terminal disease, Hepatitis C.

Most people think Hepatitis C is something you get from drinking too much. Really, people don't have a clue.

The wedding was an exquisite and gracious three days of ceremonial bliss. The following morning the newlyweds took several of us out for a late brunch. This was the first time I'd paid an ATM three dollars for a forty-dollar transaction.

This event is in this book because my ability to function was in the stage of deterioration, a stage where you gravitate from here to the other side.

I was on a quest to purchase the main item which leads to recovery: live cell Thymus extracted from the thymus gland of calves.

This wedding, a celebration of life, was a most joyous event. One that reminded me of the story about Jesus and his first holy miracle of turning water to wine at the marriage in Canaan of Galilee. It was the first wedding I remember where the bride and groom maintained composure at all times.

Thank you Kathy and Chris, for the time of my life, and may love be with you all of your life. Great and gracious to thee for sharing this blessed time with me. To this day I remember the date. I kept the napkins and matches from beside my plate. Kathy and Chris, September 7, 1996, a trio of days filled with bliss

Chapter Six

1996

It was yesterday that I attended my appointment. The one I had waited for, for over a year. This was partly because it took months to get in but mostly because it took years to save enough money to pay for the appointment.

I anxiously drove down Pacific Coast Highway to Wilshire Boulevard where I encountered massive lunchtime traffic that consisted of all classes of misfits, frantically roaming the streets at lunch hour. I was angry, having traversed this town many years earlier and knowing somewhere in my brain that I knew exactly where I was and where I was going.

I thought I missed the turn. I was confused, due to toxins in my blood interfering with my brain function. I was sort of not all there and not in control. The minutes ticked off. I was angry, but steeped in high anticipation. I was elated at the prospects of attaining information, from the greatest possible source on the planet earth, about the disease that was killing me.

Yes, here I was, after long anticipation, waiting to absorb every great morsel of healing news that would be entering my ears. I was ready to absorb all of this unknown, invigorating medical advice about to be bestowed on me by the esteemed highest of the high _ _ _-_ _ _ -_ _ _ _ M.D. Hepatologist. He was a hepatologist of the liver transplant program at Cedars Sinai Medical Center.

The waiting room was huge, larger than anything I'd ever seen. It was impeccably decorated. I only enjoyed the great magazine selections for a few short moments, and then I was whisked away into the chamber where, in only moments, I would meet the great Hepatologist.

_ _ _ _ B.S.N.,R.N., hepatology nurse took my blood pressure. It was 178/140. She was sweet, very nice and gentle.

Then the Hepatologist entered.

He was about my age, seemed uptight and asked questions for about an hour; questions he said were very important.

He attempted to lead me to believe Interferon was the only possible route.

He said, and he said it four or five times in one paragraph, "The one thing I dislike more than anything else is treating a patient who is intelligent and well read; and you are intelligent and well read." He also said there was not anything he could tell me to do or not to do, nothing I should or shouldn't eat, nor anything I should or should not take. He said that after my test results were back, he would call me and discuss them with me.

I ask him his opinion of a high albumin count and its effects on the immune system and explained to him what

I had recently learned about albumin. He stated "That is the most ridiculous thing I have ever heard". This visit cost me $788.00. Oh yeah.

I came home, called Patty, and then directed my efforts toward finding a source for live cell Thymus on the Internet.

Chapter Seven

Hepatitis C Researcher

I began taking live cell Thymus several months prior to my visit to the Hepatologist, along with a regimen of other items, many of which I had never heard, that were prescribed by Dr. John Finnegan, N.D. (Naturopathic Medicine).

Reishi mushrooms, real "shrooms", not a pill, and drinking a tea that took me six hours to make. I made the tea two or three times a week.

I boiled milk thistle seed and made a tea from it too. No tea bags, no pills from a bottle, but real things from real plants. They were time consuming events, but hey, this is my life. Modern medicine gave it all they had and modern medicine failed!

There was also lipoic acid. My brother told me about a doctor he had heard on a radio show in Washington who treated Hepatitis C with vitamin C injections combined with lipoic acid, a vitamin co-factor. To my understanding, lipoic acid is something that complements vitamin C in the body. I took lipoic acid plus two to three Thymus capsules two or three times a day, and many other new and interesting items, not vitamins, but food in pill form.

I soon began to feel much better, especially on the days when I took the live cell Thymus. At first I took it twice a week. Taking it caused me to feel completely normal, health-wise that is. So I began taking it more often, and then every other day.

About three weeks after my visit to the Hepatologist, his terrific well-mannered and proper nurse (whose clothes I wanted to tear off and have wild sex with right there in the reception room) called me to inform me that most of the tests had to be redone. The liver panel was good and showed that the three indicators were three and four numbers above normal. This was a great reduction from my previous battery of blood-sucking, money-grabbing analysis.

One year later and I was broke. I had exhausted all assets seeking out the secret and expensive health knowledge buried in catacombs. Now I began to understand why.

I made an appointment with the great Hepatitis C research doctor, UCLA's best. The researcher of the great, noble and respected UCLA Medical Center, a leader in the world today. A teaching institution that passed on the great tendencies of arrogance, the beliefs they're paid to find and make sure that not anything else is said.

I drove directly to the UCLA Medical Center, passing by the welfare office on Veterans Street, where two years earlier I tried to get some help with the expensive and deadly Interferon. Paying my five dollars at the parking center I, confused and disoriented, inquired at the information center for them to direct my sickly being to the entrance of the digestive disease center. When I arrived there I was whisked away to a hallway, blood pressure taken, and then weighed on a scale in kilos. I had to translate the kilos into pounds for the nurse because she could not read the chart. I was asked the usual questions: what drugs do you take and what medicines? I began to list my herb intake. She just wrote herbs.

After waiting for about ten minutes and having read and researched every item in the "vacuum", a beautiful student doctor came into the room. She was nice, asked the usual questions: were my feces black, etc? She was about to leave, told me the "big chief" would be in soon, and oh yes, she needed to perform a prostate exam on me. She said, "Please pull down your pants." I thought, "Sure baby, how about a quickie while we're at it?" Hepatitis C is a blood born disease so "lets go". She really laid on the grease. Truly she should specialize in prostrate examinations because her finger was so small, and she was really good at it.

The Hepatitis C research doctor entered. All I could think of was the grease soaking through my pants. I was going to have to walk out of there, and people were going to think I went in my pants.

The doctor said a few words, nothing remarkable, and then sent me to the lab for blood work. In between, I was fleeced for $188.00 plus lab fees of $360.00, for total of $548 for this.

The blood work technicians were like students, and certainly from a different economic class than at Cedars Medical Center. Rich Israelis mostly occupy Cedars, truly a safe place to be. UCLA is more like school. Nobody there seemed completely confident, except for the Hepatitis C research doctor and he knew it all.

The "blood sucking" technician ripped a hole in my arm, causing my deodorant to fail and the perspiration to flow, all because she would not listen to me. Finally, after a near death experience, she got help. I was bandaged, treated for shock and sent home.

A few months went by and two days before each of my appointments, someone called and left a message. I would call back and change the appointment to a few weeks later as I had no money. I've always had a hard time making doctors' appointments unless I had money to pay for them. Someday, I might need a good mechanic, and I wouldn't want to be denied one because I failed to pay.

It's May 29th, and I drove past Mezzaluna restaurant, briefly contemplating getting away with murder. I entered the medical center parking facility and behold, one of the "Japanese invaders" at the tollbooth asked, "Have you been here before?" "Yes", I responded and she said, "You mean I don't have to give you a long dissertation about where you are going?" Not unless you can elaborate on how to get to heaven.

I got on the wrong elevator with an older gentleman, and it only stopped at parking lot levels. We, after much button pushing, arrived right where we had started. He got excited and stayed right by my side, as if I were the messiah. Finally, I escaped from him by sneaking past a wheelchair in another very crowded elevator.

I got off on the wrong floor; well the stairs were cool. The waiting room offered a day old LA Times food section about Nepalese cactus, something I grew at my Rancho Loco, Malibu. When you cook them they're really slimy like ochre.

I went down the hallway, where a young lady took my blood pressure. She said, "Let me have your arm." I said, "Where would you like it?" She wasn't sure how to respond. However, she knew how to read a kilo scale, and I went off to the same "vacuum" I examined on my prior visit.

A young male Japanese doctor; a tall, confident and pleasant-mannered fellow, came right in and immediately began reviewing my blood test. He said I was in perfect health, and I should see a psychiatrist. I requested a look at my blood tests, and sure enough, they were perfect. They were not just perfect, but absolutely perfect, from top to bottom. He took my test results back, said the doctor would be in soon and he was. The great and all knowing Hepatitis C research doctor said, "Mr. Wright, you are well. You no longer have any sign of disease. We could not find any Hepatitis C virus in your system. Your blood test numbers were perfect. I'm going to refer you to a psychiatrist." I said, "I guess my live cell Thymus worked. Pretty cool, huh?" His response, "some people think Elvis is still alive." I then tried to inform him of my two thousand dollar a month romance with various herbs that had cured me. He said again,

"Some people believe Elvis is alive and has two heads. All that stuff is crap. It has absolutely no use whatsoever. Stop wasting your money on junk and take some of it for a few visits to a good Psychiatrist. You will feel three hundred percent better. He will give you a little pill that won't hurt your liver and you won't believe how good you'll feel."

I further attempted to inform him of my herbal intake as cautiously as possible. I felt it necessary for him to understand that I was, in fact, healed from this terminal virus by using herbs, supplements and foods. This virus that afflicts five to fifteen million Americans. Perhaps they too could benefit from my expensive research and discovery. After all, he was a research doctor, an Interferon research doctor. Needless to say, he refused to even listen to the facts.

In my case, I had documents from several doctors over a six-year period showing liver numbers from various labs before, during and after Interferon. I had documented proof that after Interferon, I still had Hepatitis C, and that the numbers had begun to rise.

After a year and a half of herbal remedies, available to everyone on the planet, I was well. No Hepatitis C was detectable, and the American medical machine does not want you to know.

I was paying this man cash for his time, and all he did was make Elvis Jokes. I was appalled.

Now I clearly saw why American medicine could not cure the common cold. Because no one was funding it. They just fund things that suppressed it. If they cured it, the money machine would stop. Sounds unbelievable, doesn't it? I have been in the "chamber of the gods" and they only have allegiance to their pharmaceutical funders rather than to the patient and his or her welfare.

I was thoroughly appalled. We live in society where doctors deny reality, and only adhere to their agendas. Though difficult to believe, I experienced it time and again as I dealt with Hepatitis C.

During the Hepatitis C research doctor's dissertation of Elvis jokes, he claimed herb use was not documented. The reason it wasn't was because people, such as he, refused to even hear about it.

Somehow, it seemed to me that a man in his position could be saving thousands and even millions of lives from years of immeasurable suffering and prolonged agonizing deaths, if what worked on me worked on others. He was in a position to cause that to happen.

Instead, what I learned from my long journey was that one Naturopathic Medicine Dr. in Malibu and one Chiropractor; two people, who are looked upon with skepticism, knew that their efforts and my extensive research had worked on me.

Chapter Eight

Media Hype Chapter Seven

Recently I heard that Bob Dole refused contributions from gay Americans. I respected this, not because they were gay, but because they were stupid.

Let it be known, that Auto Immune Deficiency Syndrome (AIDS) is a virus that is almost always, at this point in time, transmitted by sexual contact. Here and now, let us remind ourselves that yes, there are a few who have been terrorized by this infirmity through blood transfusions. I am not referring to those unfortunate people.

Human Immunodeficiency Virus (HIV) and AIDS afflict people who have committed illicit deeds. They've had some form of sex with someone other than their partner, wife, husband or companion; otherwise they could not get it. Unless they had a threesome, or were "swappers", which I suppose if you are a realist and somewhat perverted, is O.K. but nevertheless condemned by God.

Why is there so much media hype about AIDS? It's a disease that worldwide six thousand people a day get through illicit, immoral and indecent sex. Illicit sex, condemned by society, but practiced by many homosexuals, a large and organized voting block.

Between 1985 and 1998 there have been 688,200 cases of AIDS reported and 410,800 deaths reported from AIDS in the United States, according to the Centers for Disease Control and Prevention. 17,047 people died from AIDS in 1998, down from 21,222 in 1997. The Center for Disease Control and Prevention states that 4,000,000 Americans are infected with Hepatitis C and 2.7 million are chronically infected. The Los Angles Times reports that at least one half million people in California have Hepatitis C and at least 41% of the prison population is infected. The misery, the suffering, the fear and expense for people with Hepatitis C is experienced by millions of Americans while AIDS is only affecting a small portion in comparison. While the number of AIDS related deaths has dropped significantly over the last few years, the number of deaths from Hepatitis is expected to triple over the next ten years.

Over ninety percent of people with HCV caught their destiny from a blood transfusion, other hospital procedures or from dental work. I recently noticed that during the annual HCV conference in Chicago, the media hype liked to emphasize that HCV is a sexually transmitted disease (STD). Hepatitis C is not an STD!

It's true that doctors like to say this during their conferences, but do not mention at all the fact that most of us got this "great reward" in doctors' offices and hospitals.

As a result of the way we have received Hepatitis C, we are a random section of the populace, not a clear and distinct voting block. Politicians want the support of a distinct voting block so gays and their disease benefit.

In the United States HCV doesn't have the organized group effort that they do in Canada. It's truly random. You are in a traffic accident, go to the hospital, receive blood and die from HCV. You want some perky "tits", so you go to a plastic surgeon, who transforms your "droopers" to "mammoth mammaries", and you pay with your life.

There are those who received their reward from needles by injecting their good times, not knowing that they were playing Russian roulette with a yet unknown disease. It was unknown until discovered in 1989, a mere decade ago.

As most Americans have heard, HCV is a celebrity disease: Mickey Mantle, David Crosby, Naomi Judd and Larry Hagman are just a few who have suffered from Hepatitis C and its complications.

As a result of public outcry about giving preference to celebrities, the National Transplant Association changed its rules. All Hepatitis C patients are now considered third state recipients. That means that if you have Hepatitis C, you are probably not going to receive a liver.

The Association's reasoning is that the new liver will also be infected by the disease that is carried in the persons blood, and they will eventually die anyway, (unless they and you read my book). A person in a traffic accident who needs a liver, and wasn't drunk while driving, will get a liver before a person with Hepatitis C.

If you were in a traffic accident that originally caused you to get the disease, where lies the morality of the events that generated the new guidelines?

For those of you reading this book, you probably won't need a new liver. I have not researched this much because I could never afford a liver transplant. The government won't give me Medi-Cal coverage, so I know I will never have a new liver. Still, the beaurocrats and doctors responsible for the current guidelines have their heads in the clouds.

I want the whole world to see and know of the horrendous injustices created due to the voting blocks reported by the media. I want the world to understand that the search for a cure appears to be more aggressive, based on the greed of politicians for their voting blocks. Also doctors are hiding from their responsibility of spreading HCV in the United States.

When the whole picture is examined it causes one to look down and sadly shake his or her head, while the gays, politicians and doctors are saluting the flag.

In fifteen Asian countries, experiments are being conducted that are producing excellent results in curing Hepatitis C. Products used in these experiments cannot even be purchased in the United States.

Chapter Nine

PATS Report

About a year ago a letter from the Hepatitis Foundation International (HFI) found its way to the "stomach" of my baseball bat-beaten mailbox. Enclosed was a form with a space for my phone number. If I signed and returned it to 30 Sunrise Terrace, Cedar Grove, CA, I could be put on something called the PATS Report. This report contains a list of names and phone numbers of other unfortunates with the same infirmity.

The list arrived. It was on yellow paper with black ink. It had first names, phone numbers, city, and Hepatitis interest; a clever way to discern who had B or C or both B and C. After scanning through the list, I decided to call some people in cities closest to me. B from Canoga Park was my first call. He answered and was right up front with me. He said he had done a lot of speed and figured he got Hepatitis from dirty needles. He didn't know for sure. He told me that his son also was infected with the C virus. His words about the doctors he and his son have supported intersected with my pool of disgust, the depth of which amazed even me.

It was October 18, 1998, and the bastards still didn't get it.

B told me that his doctor told him not to worry as long as it didn't bother him.

Why does advice such as that cost hundreds of thousands of dollars? It's for education resulting in the capital letters accompanying a person's name, letters that lend distinguishing results such as Dr., or M.D., or Ph.D.

College, for me, was some drink, lots of sex and running naked across the college campus. It also was fast sports cars along with a degree of ethical behavior that resulted in what I'm putting on paper.

Truly I wish that I had spent more serious effort at almost everything in life, because women have really turned out to be over-rated. At least many of the ones I've known.

The silent killer is working on B and his son. A simple change in diet and a few herbs would make a vast difference in the progression of their silent killer.

B had a fax machine so I proceeded to fax him a copy of my "bad blood" test results, a copy of my liver biopsy and the results of two other blood tests. One from September 22, 1998, and one from April 10, 1997; both perfect, no RNA viral infection of Hepatitis C. I included a copy of my herb list and diet.

A while later B called back. This time he was filled with enthusiasm. He wanted to know where to get the items. I shared all my secrets with him. I shared a list of things that cost me thousands of dollars to compile. I did this just so he could get well.

Here lies my need to tell the whole world about how I got well. While what I did may not cure everyone, I believe that the research I reviewed for this book supports that it should work on most humans the way it worked on me. Good luck B and remain on my program.

M from Melview: "I'm tired. I can't remember what my doctors

said. I've taken to the Lord. God will deal with it. Never would I take something, unless my doctor told me to."

She asked, "Are you a doctor?" "No," I replied.

She said, "Well, you should be ashamed of yourself for making believe you can cure something. Shame on you."

This woman I couldn't help.

If she would read her Bible, she would find in the Old Testament that God said he provided all the herbs to cure all the infirmities that would affect man.

She did mention that heavy donations to her church were sure to save her. Certainly, I didn't disagree with giving to the church. I know God can (and sometimes does) heal.

When I had cancer I went to church every Sunday. I attended prayer meetings and was baptized in a nearby swimming pool. My name was printed alongside Michael Landon's in the church paper each week asking for prayer.

One fine day, the preacher preached a whole sermon about how badly he needed a clear plastic pulpit to stand behind. It would signify and bring power to our small gathering of born-again believers.

It was a time when I was very sick, and I was taken in by his request. I asked the preacher how much it would cost, and promptly wrote a check for five hundred dollars.

A few months later that fine, clear plastic pulpit arrived and that preacher was behind it with his fly down! I was in the front row and was so embarrassed. After about two hours he finally discovered his fly was down and then spent two more hours disciplining the congregation for allowing him to carry on and not tell him.

A few months later that preacher bought a washing machine for a tribe of nuns in Africa, a place where they had no laundry detergent, hot water or even electricity.

Shortly after, he ran off to South America with a good-looking girl from the choir. He left his wife, his friends and everything else, except the money. I guess he needed that money to carry out the Lord's work?

Please don't get me wrong here, I love God and know he created me. I could not be, if not for him. A strange thought just occurred to me. How many doctors do you know who believe in God?

Basically, in my pursuit to help the people on my yellow list, I've encountered three distinct types of responses: the interested, the disinterested and most of all the "I wouldn't do anything unless my doctor told me to do it." I'd be dead now if I followed that shallow train of thought. I suppose those were the people who voted for Bill Clinton.

That one item, I wouldn't do anything unless my doctor told me to do it, flowed across all the testimony of most people on PATS Report.

Their doctors didn't know how to cure hepatitis C. And of course they didn't bother to do any other research in order to save the lives of their patients. This still baffles me. Was I a mutant? Perhaps I've missed some important dose of civilized behavior along the way. I was reminded of a movie, Soilent Green, where people just walked right into this huge machine that turned them into food. Only Charlton Heston rebelled and exposed what was going on. Was Timmy Leary right? Did that acid trip I took when I was twenty really open my mind?

Chapter Ten

The Letter

For those of you who believe that my brain is permanently damaged - which at this time I have no quarrel with - I bring you more evidence of the used-car-salesmanship mentality that these key people at the pinnacle of this pillar of crap, called Fight Against Hepatitis C. I bring you their lack of interest and their blatant disregard for the facts about which they are supposed to be inquiring.

I have included a portion from the newsletter, *Alert*, published by the Hepatitis Foundation International (HFI). This organization constantly sent me material, requesting cash donations to support its yacht and Rolls Royce payments. The issue included is dated, Fall 1998.

HFI'S CEO Serves on NIH Alternative Medicine Planning Committee

Thelma King Thiel. Chair and CEO of HFL has been invited to serve on the complementary and Alternative Medicine (CAM) Planning Committee at the National Institute of Health "I'm pleased to be representing patients and HFI in this effort to evaluate the safety and effectiveness of complementary and alternative treatments for hepatitis and other chronic liver disease,." Said Mrs. Thiel. "The fact that Congress has appropriated an additional $50 million to the Office of Alternative Medicine is very encouraging."

The CAM Planning Committee has been formed to assess knowledge of complementary and alternative medicine for chronic liver disease, focusing on the availability of scientific evidence for efficacy and safety; to identify and prioritize research needs that will fully define the efficacy and safety of CAM for liver diseases; and to form a consensus on the state-of-the-art of CAM for liver disease. The committee hopes to disseminate the consensus to both the medical and lay communities through (a) the publication of the conference proceedings and an executive summary, and (b) publication of lay informational materials disseminated through NJDDK clearinghouse and lay foundations.

Reading this Newsletter excerpt was the highlight of my recent existence. I was well and I tested HCV non-detected. Immediately I called Thelma King Thiel and spoke with her secretary. She informed me that her boss would love to speak with me about my ordeal and cure; however, her boss was currently on a conference call and would call me back as soon as she finished.

During my conversation with the secretary, I explained my battle and eventual cure and that UCLA had declared me Hepatitis free. She asked me to fax some material so Ms. Thiel could have a look as they were very interested. She gave me the fax number and within minutes, I faxed her the following documents.

To: Thelma King Thiel

I read last night that you were invited to serve on the (CAM) planning committee.

I was infected with Hep C in 1979 from a blood transfusion.

It was finally diagnosed in 1994.

I cured it with alternative medicine.

I would like to discuss this with you because I believe it could help many people and most doctors. Those I've described my program to, do not take me seriously.

Thank You,

Lloyd Wright

Surgeon: D. MD

Date of Surgery: 12/16/94

Date Accessioned: 12/16/94

Blocks: 1

Recuts:

Stains:

Specimen (s):

Liver biopsy

OR Consultation:

Gross Description:

The specimen is labeled Lloyd Wright- UTSD liver Biopsy. It consists of two thread like pieces of soft pink-white tissue measuring 0.7 cm in length and 1.5 cm. In length and averaging 0.1 cm. In diameter or less. The tissue has a stripped appearance. TE-1. RLR: do

Diagnosis, including microscopic examination:

Chronic Hepatitis consistent with hepatitis C; UTSD liver biopsy (see microscopic description and Comment).

a. The sections show hepatitis tissue with moderate to marked chronic lymphocyte inflammation that is predominantly periportal. Focally lymphocytes percolate out into the hepatic lobules in the sinusoids. There is mild to focally moderate steatosis with predominantly large droplet fatty change. In some of the portal areas, the bile ducts appear attenuated by the inflammatory process. The features are consistent with hepatitis C infection. Definitive piecemeal necrosis is not seen. Mallory's hyaline is not seen. Special stains for iron reveal minimal focal positive staining involving hepatocytes. Special stains for connective tissue reveal a mild to moderate periportal fibrosis with a few portal areas showing tendrils of bridging fibrosis. No regenerative nodules of cirrhosis are seen.

Comment: The Tissue block will be sent for hepatic iron analysis at MLN. Results will be forwarded as soon as they are received.

Completion Date: 12/20/94

RLR:sg

CAL Clinical Laboratories	Patient: Wright, Lloyd Sex: M Age: 40 Lab # 4783255
Date of Specimen: 01/30/91	Time Reported: 5:54 AM

Hematology	**Results**	**Units**	**Ref. Range**
WBC	6.38	Thous/CMM	4.30-11.0
RBC	5.18	M/CMM	4.7-6.1
HGB	16.1	GM %	14-18
HCT	46.7	%	42-52
MCV	90.2	CU Micron	77-102
MCH	31.1	M MCGMS	27-32
MCHC	34.5	%	32-36
Platelet Count	273	Thous/CMM	130-400
Neut	67.3	%	50-75
Lymphs	26.8	%	20-40
Monos	4.1	%	0-10
Eos	1.6	%	0-5
Baso	.2	%	0-3
Biochemistry – A			
ALKP'tase, Total	115	MU/ML	30-115
LDH Total	234	MU/ML	100-250
AST	**210**	MU/ML	1-41
ALT	**245**	MU/ML	0-45
GGTP	**215**	MU/ML	0-65
Total Protein Serum	8.5	GM/DL	6.0-8.5
Albumin	5.1	GM/DL	3.0-5.5
Globulin, Total	3.4	GM/DL	1.9-3.5
A/G Ration, Chemical	1.5	Ratio	1.0-2.2
Bilirubin, Total	.5	MG/DL	0-1.5
Bilirubin, Direct	.1	MG/DL	0-.4
Bilirubin, Indirect	.4	MG/DL	0-1.2

DISPLAY/PRINT RESULTS | STANDARD DISPLAY COLLECTED LAST 4 MONTHS | THU 05/29/97 0852 PAGE 01 BY LM#LDK

PATIENT ID	PATIENT NAME	SEX	AGE	UNIT/S	RM/BED	TEMP	LOCATION
219-29-02 1	WRIGHT, LLOYD	M	47				

-P TEST NAME	F RESULTS	UNITS	REF RANCE
04/10/97 1430	(COLLECTION TIME)	1527 (IN LAB TIME)	
CHEMISTRY PANEL			
CHEMISTRY PANEL COMMENT	PROFILE PERFORMED		
SODIUM,PANEL	139	mmol/L	136-146
POTASSIUM, PANEL	4.1	mmol/L	3.6-5.0
CHLORIDE,PANEL	102	mmol/L	97-110
CO2 CONTENT,PANEL	28	mmol/L	25-32
GLUCOSE,PANEL	89	mg/dL	65-110
CREATININE,PANEL	0.9	mg/dL	0.5-1.2
UREA NITROGEN, PANEL	12	mg/dL	8-20
TOTAL PROTEIN, PANEL	7.6	g/dL	6.0-8.0
ALBUMIN, PROTEIN	4.7	g/dL	3.7-4.8
PHOSPHORUS, PANEL	3.4	mg/dL	2.6-4.2
BILIRUBIN, TOTAL, PANEL	0.7	mg/dL	0.3-1.2

- TEST NAME	F RESULT	UNITS	REF RANGE
04/10/97 1430 (COLLECTION TIME)	04/10/97	1527	(IN LAB TIME)
CHEMISTRY PANEL	CONTINUED...		
ALKALINE PHOSPHATASE, PANEL	86	U/L	35-110
AST (SSGT), PANEL	23	U/L	5-50
ALT (SGPT), PANEL	12	U/L	5-50
CHOLESTEROL,PANEL	239	mg/dL	0-240
CALCIUM, PANEL	9.8	mg/dL	8.4-10.0
TSH	0.9	mIU/L	0.3-4.7

END OF REPORT

Radiation Center Date of Specimen: Time Reported: 09/22/98 4:30 AM		Patient: Wright, Lloyd Sex: M Age: 48 Spec. No. 44291763	
Test Name	**Results**	**Ref. Range**	**Units**
Basic Metabolic Panel			
Glucose	99	65-110	MG/DL
Sodium	145	135-148	ME/QL
Potassium	4	3.5-5.5	ME/QL
Chloride	102	95-107	ME/QL
CO2	26	22-34	ME/QL
BUN	19	6-25	MG/DL
Creatinine	.9	.5-1.4	MG/DL
BUN/Creatinine	21.1	10-28	Ratio
Albumin	4.5	4.1-5.4	G/DL
Bilirubin, Total	.4	.1-1.5	MG/DL
Bilirubin, Direct	.1	0-.3	MG/DL
ALK Phos, Total	**49**	30-125	U/L
AST	**21**	1-45	U/L
ALT	**14**	1-45	U/L
CBC w/Diff			
WBC	5.5	4-11	X10*3/CUM
RBC	4.54	4.2-5.5	X10*6/CUM
Hemoglobin	14.9	13-17	GraMs./DL
Hematocrit	42.9	38-50	%
MCV	94	82-97	Cubic Mic.
MCH	32.8	27-34	PicograMs.
MCHC	34.7	32-36	%
RDW	11.6	11.5-15.2	%
Platelet Count	175	150-400	XFL
MPV	8.4	5.2-11.1	0*3/CUM
Neutrophils	61	50-70	%
Lymphocytes	23	15-50	%
Monocytes	13	0-10	%
Eosinophils	2	0-5	%
Basophils	1	0-5	%

Let's go over this again. Thelma King Thiel, Chair and CEO of Hepatitis Foundation International, was invited to serve on the Complimentary and Alternative Medicine (CAM) Planning Committee at the National Institute of Health. She commented:

> I'm pleased to be representing patients and HFI in this effort to evaluate the safety and effectiveness of complimentary and alternative treatments for Hepatitis...The fact that congress has appropriated an additional $50 million to the office of Alternative medicine is very encouraging. The CAM planning committee has been formed to assess knowledge of complimentary and alternative medicine for chronic liver diseases (1).

Considering what you've just read, I faxed Ms. Thiel a brief letter stating I was cured from chronic Hepatitis C. I included a copy of my liver biopsy dated 12/16/94 as proof of my cure. The biopsy was performed at Los Robles Hospital in Thousand Oaks, California. I also included a copy of one blood test from 1/30/91, showing my AST (SGOT) Panel at 210 when it should have been between 1 and 41. My ALT (SGPT) Panel was at 245, which should have been between 0 and 45, and my GGTP at 215, which should have been in the range of 0-65. I sent a copy of the results of this test because it was easily accessible, and it showed a long period of time between tests, indicating I'd been infected for many years.

I also faxed her a copy of the results of my blood test taken on 4/10/97 at UCLA. This test showed AST

(SGOT) Panel at 23, normal range between 5-40 and ALT (SGPT) Panel at 12, normal range between 5-50. These results were better than perfect. They indicated that my liver functions were better than normal for a person of my age with my history. It was, in a word, phenomenal. Not a miracle, but the results of dedicated study and practice of what I learned.

Further, I faxed Ms.Thiel a copy of the results of a blood test taken 9/22/98, showing AST (SGOT) at 21, normal range 1-45; and ALT (SGPT) at 14, normal range 1-45. These test results were selected because they were my most recent and showed that even as I continued with my naughty habits, I continued to stay well after years had passed. These tests proved that I was cured from Hepatitis C. I've read and know first hand that this did not happen to most people who survived Interferon.

This material should arouse the interests of anyone, especially a foundation determined to help find a solution for this disease. However, it didn't seem to interest Ms. Thiel. I thought it would because of her new position. Please absorb her letter to me dated December 30,1998, on the following page. Read it two or three times and then think about your fifty million in tax money that went to support Alternative Medicine. Think about your health. If you have Hepatitis C, wouldn't you want to know how I became well?

HEPATITIS FOUNDATION
INTERNATI0NAL

December 30, 1998

Mr. Lloyd Wright
Malibu, CA 90265

Dear Mr. Wright:

Thank you for writing. I'm delighted that you are in good shape.

Fortunately, recent research reports indicate that many people with biopsies like yours will not advance to serious liver disease but will remain healthy carriers. This is very encouraging news.

Good luck and stay well.

Sincerely,

Thelma King Thiel
Chairman and Chief
Executive Officer

You've hopefully digested the fact that these people in high places just don't give a damn. I shall continue to show you that Hepatitis C is being handled in a fashion which defies belief.

Naomi Judd, a truly fascinating personality, often referred to as "The Queen of Country".

The American Liver Foundation (ALF) sent out thousands of copies of letters written by Naomi. She described her feelings when she was diagnosed with Hepatitis C and how Hepatitis C had changed her life. She described her daily awareness of the "spirit, mind, body connection", and how she has dedicated her life to finding a cure for Hepatitis and other liver diseases.

By the end of the first page you are undoubtedly about to sob; but by page two, the tears flow as Naomi relates to you how her first course of treatment with Interferon in 1990 didn't work.

She writes:

> I was so sick and so scared. . . I thought I was going to die. In 1996 I started a second course of Interferon treatment and, when this was finished one year later, my doctor told me that the virus could no longer be found in my blood. I was so happy. I still can't stop thanking God. However, many people do not respond to therapy, so I am dedicating my life to finding a cure because there is so much more we need to know . . . and do (2).

I wondered what "and do" means? She knows the cure? Could it be that the liver foundation didn't want her to say it?

Naomi goes on for about five more paragraphs hyping Interferon, the research of the American Liver Foundation, hoping for more treatment options, and begging you to send your hard earned money to this callous organization.

She pleads, "Please join me in accepting that responsibility and with your generous contribution, creating a 'Campaign of Hope' that will support the essential work of the American Liver Foundation."

Well Naomi Judd, National Honorary Spokesperson, you are a most elegant and remarkable person. However, as I see it you speak with forked tongue, or perhaps your Hepatitis C caused a lapse in your memory?

Let's go back to January 1998, Issue 21 of *Alternative Medicine Digest*:

> Naomi spent the next six years looking into a range of alternative medicines. A program of nutritional and herbal supplements strengthened her immune system and lent support to her beleaguered liver. She takes (and the article goes on to describe much of what I did: vitamins, milk thistle, thymus glandular extract from calves). Naomi's liver enzyme levels, which had gone up again after the Interferon cycle ended, dropped to within the normal range after she added the thymus glandulars to her program (3).

It's remarkable what you can find out there if you've got the money and the energy to find it. Money alone won't do it. Naomi and I have had a very similar group of occurrences, based on what I've read in the Alternative Medicine Digest article.

I am very pleased that she is well, but it does bother me that she sells Interferon with what appears to be great enthusiasm and leaves out the genuine pieces of healing news, for you to find elsewhere. But the ALF probably just pays her to say what they want her to say, not necessarily the whole truth.

Hopefully Naomi will go back and demand that the ALF allow her to tell the entire story. You owe it to everyone who has this dreaded disease.

Unfortunately, this dirt and corruption persists throughout the entire spectrum wherever there is a dollar to be made.

Chapter Eleven

Dark Ages

Ethics, morality, they no longer exist. It's as if we were strung out on a long acid trip mixed with a pound of good Afghani hash and a few buttons of peyote. Then there appeared before us a giant eraser, and we wiped ourselves clean.

It's all about image. Image is all there is. Whether it's you, corporations, the great renowned learning institutions or the corner store. It's just image. There is no substance. Doctors are a prime example of this illusion. They even want you to imagine yourself well. An article in the fall 1998 issue of *Hepatitis Alert*, titled "Placebos & Positive Beliefs Help Healing" states, "An enthusiastic physician who provides encouragement that the treatment will work provides hope and optimism to patients" (1).

This statement indicates to me that if I have a good doctor and he tells me that the poison known as INTERFERON ALFA-2B RECOMBINANT will cure me, and I believe him, that I will be just fine. What is this, the Dark Ages?

We, Americans, are the first known people ever to inhabit the earth, who feed our most precious meat source a strict diet of chicken manure and "40 billion pounds a year of slaughterhouse wastes such as blood, bone, viscera, as well as the remains of millions of euthanized cats and dogs passed along by veterinarians and animal shelters" (4). This means that America's pets are and have been for years, used as cattle food. Our pets, as well as ROAD KILLS, dehydrated food garbage, fats emptied from restaurant fryers and grease traps, cement kiln dust, newsprint, cardboard, hog manure and yes we even feed our cows human sewage sludge (4). Truly America is the greatest country on earth. The reason you all believe that is because you are literally full of manure.

Our prestigious learning institutions and great medical facilities even dump their cadavers, mixed with toxic waste, into the Santa Monica Bay.

These cadavers were the remains of the great and noble people who donated their bodies to science to further the study of all things that plague humans. In return, they were promised a proper burial.

In the name of the almighty dollar, The University of California at Los Angeles (UCLA), and no doubt other institutions, burned these cadavers slightly and tossed the remains in the bay (5).

An LA Times article documented this practice:

> Without admitting guilt UCLA has agreed to pay $49,500 and strengthen its medical waste practices to settle charges that it violated the law in disposing of human remains at its medical school. UCLA and the State Department of Health

> Services said that they were happy with the agreement, which stems from an October 1993 incident in which the skipper of a burial-at-sea service accidentally broke open a box of ashes that UCLA had wanted dumped into the Santa Monica Bay. The box contained cremated remains of cadavers used by UCLA Medical School, but also contained pieces of glass and surgical equipment (5).

In this article, the skipper of the boat and one state investigator said that hair was also found on some of the remains and rubber stoppers were still in some bottles, "indicating a possible low temperature in the incinerator that burned the remains" (5). In the settlement UCLA agreed to close its on-campus crematorium and send all cadavers used by its medical school, off campus for disposal and burial. A Department of Health Services Investigator, named McGurk, indicated that the fact that UCLA was a student and taxpayer supported institution figured into the monetary settlement. What we didn't read, but must know, is that there was no doubt a huge profit stuck in the pockets of those few individuals at the medical school who carried out these illegal, evil deeds. Surely there were large bills for proper burial, and big costs for proper cremation. The manner in which the entire incident just disappeared, indicates big payoffs. UCLA teaches ethics in more places than its classrooms.

What we as a society have become is in the strictest sense phenomenal. I've been trying to tell people about the unethical operations of many renowned institutions for years. People think I'm nuts when I tell them that the American cows' diet is chicken manure. I've seen those seventy-five foot high mounds of mixed rations on cattle ranches in many places around the U.S. We are in DENIAL!

"Toxic heavy metal: arsenic, lead, cadmium, and mercury can collect in organs and tissues of cattle. Effects on humans who eat tainted beef are uncertain" (6). However, what we eat has a lot to do with our causes of dying. One in three of us will be greeted with cancer, and eating meat from cows that are fed a chicken manure diet doesn't help us.

Who is stupid here? We can't afford to feed ourselves, or the world, so we have lapsed into a state that can not continue. A great decline will surely take place in order to readjust our behavior.

Since the sixties, I have been listening to individuals tell me red meat is bad. Many people express all sorts of unusual effects from eating cows e.g. feeling dirty from eating meat . . . I believe that many of us are sensitive to red meat because of what the host animal was fed.

If you concur that it is the development of these unethical practices in the name of saving money, then it becomes easy to see that we cannot afford to feed ourselves. We have become futile in our attempts to feed ourselves.

Our farmers have been overfarming the same land for hundreds of years. In most cases, farmers are only replacing three chemicals to the earth: nitrogen, potash and phosphate. This has been practiced throughout the last half of the 20th century. There are hundreds of known trace minerals, nutrients, salts, and probably unknown quantities of other elements that have been depleted from our soils, and these elements are no longer in our food.

The government tells us we are living longer, healthier lives. They say we eat better than any humans before, and that our medical technology is the best in the world.

I haven't heard any news recently about the righteous. We can't say God in a public school, and Jesus Christ has become a swear word. People claim they're spiritual, when they only gather a little here and a little there, and then combine these "littles" in their minds to equal spiritual.

Our lives are overburdened with getting here and getting there. We've developed "always being late" as socially proper. I hate to suggest this, but I'm going to; we have developed into a "herd" culture. I wonder if it has anything to do with what we eat?

As my eyes see, Americans are becoming uglier and uglier, except for those fortunate enough to be blessed with the qualities of stealing tons of bucks one way or another and spending them on a great plastic surgeon. Although, I've noticed that even after surgery, they really didn't feel as good as they looked.

I ponder how many of those manufactured beauties may die early because of the tainted blood they received from transfusions or the unsanitary instruments that were used in the operating room.

Things as common as having your children's teeth straightened or cavities filled have no doubt created many cases of Hepatitis C.

Hepatitis C is a deadly virus that is able to *hide* inside the liver cells.

Because of this, the virus is able to survive the immune systems' attack.

Macrophages and Kupffer cells are activated in the liver by the immune system to release chemicals to destroy the virus. The liver cells are exposed and become the unintended victim. Cirrhosis and cell death follows.

Our government, various liver agencies and doctors want us to believe that there is no group of people who have Hepatitis C. They don't want the power of a group. They want you to believe there is no GROUP of people who have Hepatitis C. That it is just random people unfortunate enough to have received a tainted blood transfusion. Blood transfusions are by far the number one culprit, but intravenous drug users and gays and lesbians have a higher incident of Hepatitis C than the general population.

However, it has come to my attention that at least ten percent, and possibly twice that number, of our veterans are infected (7).

Dr. Teresa Wright, Chief of Gastroenterology at the San Francisco VA Medical Center says, "Hepatitis C is the one nobody talks about". Dr. Wright claims that the Hepatitis C virus goes into hiding for years while it quietly works on the liver. "Eventually the result is cirrhosis or liver failure which, without a transplant, is fatal!" (7). Dr. Wright also noted that ten percent of the patients admitted to the VA Medical Center, for whatever reason, carry Hepatitis C in their blood. At least eighty percent of all those who contract the virus develop a chronic infection (7).

There are many people out there with minds, in contrast to the vacuums of the Federal Drug Administration (FDA) and its whole group of followers. It seems that the FDA, as well as the doctors in America, feel they need to create cures. They have concocted a whole new line of chemistry with really great side effects. It brings you to a near death experience, trying to kill whatever it is that is killing you, so you can survive in a seriously impaired state.

It would be wrong of me to simply stop with the feeding and eating of cows. You may, if you believe what you've been told, decide to eat fish instead; and think you'll be safer. You decide you are going to board a fishing vessel and go out and catch your own. Let the light be shed. I have a neighbor, Andy. He is a salmon fisherman. In recent years the number of salmon has plummeted, and their size is approximately one third smaller than it was just a few years ago.

Salmon swim up stream to spawn. There are many fish hatcheries up many streams. Agencies sponsored by the U.S. government are attempting to increase the number of this slippery little fish and its size. Because of the use of all sorts of growth hormones the salmon has lost much of its color. Now they're feeding them dye as well, in order to give these mutants the color of the lost race.

Occurrences of human interference are not simply limited to salmon. This sort of human tampering is being done all over the U.S. Human interference with nature produces terrible unknowns.

Ever fly over Los Angeles and land at LAX? Don't look down! If you do, you will see, for as miles and miles, structures created by people for people, tens of thousands of them. They all use toilets several times each and every day. All this human waste, along with a multitude of other toxic chemicals, is pumped into the sea. Not just Los Angeles, but along most every coast in the world, and guess what those little fish eat? Makes you sick, doesn't it?

Back when "King" Richard Nixon reigned, his "think tank" determined that the number one problem facing the world was not nuclear war, but overpopulation.

In America, it appears we are attempting to deal with overpopulation on several fronts: growing food with waste, slaughtering babies before they are born and allowing people to die who could be saved. The FDA doesn't want to hear anything about alternative sources such as the healing power of herbs.

"And God said, 'Behold I have given you every herb bearing seed, which is upon the face of all the

earth, and every tree, in which is the fruit of a tree yielding seed; to you it shall be for meat.'" (8)

News Flash! February 12, 1999, 10:30 am KNX news radio reports: "The FDA has approved radiation treatment of meat to kill bacteria." Isn't that what we used to kill the Japanese in WWII? The FDA probably does not know that radiation isn't selective about what it kills. It will probably just turn meat into a glowing fiber.

You can imagine the headlines of the future:

Meat-Packing Company Over-amps Meat!

300,000 Die as a Result of Radiation Poisoning!

Several years after this, Americans will no longer be reproducing, cattle farmers will be broke and cattle experts will no longer exist.

I am in a quandary. This process of radiation is not news to me. It just simply never occurred anywhere in my brain that this group of fools who are going to do this could possibly be that stupid. It reminds me of those commercials on the Ed Sullivan show, "BETTER LIVING THROUGH CHEMISTRY".

What is even more preposterous is that the poor unfortunate and misguided don't believe cows eat chicken manure, and don't care if they do. They don't even care because they are not convinced that this is true of "their" meat. The consequences of this apathy are beyond imagination. Future headlines for many years to come surely will reflect on such decisions as "bombing" our meat with radiation or feeding cows waste.

Part of most everything you eat, drink, smoke, snort or inject goes into or through your liver. It is the largest organ in your body and performs over twelve hundred functions.

If your liver is sick, the very first thing you must decide is; do I consume things that will surely kill my liver or do I only allow things into my liver that will not jeopardize its condition and will nourish it and help it rebuild?

Obviously, a price will be paid by any creature, human or otherwise, that eats food not intended for it, or that was not itself nourished on original food for *it*. The representations produced by laboratory analyses of the content of food, are misleading for determining the needs of living organisms in the real world (9).

Part II

The Remedy

Chapter Twelve

Milk Thistle

It was Naomi Judd from whom I learned about milk thistle. I began taking this remarkable, ancient remedy immediately and never stopped. You can acquire it in most health food stores, and it is offered in a variety of forms. Some are combined with artichoke leaves, licorice and dandelion root extract, etc. Among the best of these products are Hepastat™ and Hepata Trope™ (refer to appendix B for a list of ingredients).

I use the organic seeds, simmer them for two hours and then drink the tea iced. It is also important to take at least 1000 mg. of milk thistle per day in addition to the tea, as silymarin is not water-soluble. There are other active ingredients in milk thistle that are important but, unfortunately, most of them are eliminated from the processed capsule form. This is why I recommend the tea as well. I've reviewed many articles and studies on milk thistle and hope that some of them will find their way to all those liver doctors who told me there was nothing I could take to help my liver regenerate.

For centuries, dating back to Roman and Greek civilizations, milk thistle has been known and used as an antidote for poisoning, including snake bites. Milk thistle's derivative, silymarin is now considered medicine's most important antidote to poisoning by the mushroom toxins a-amintin and phalloidin.

Cited as one of the oldest known herbal medicines, milk thistle, part of the daisy family, is a relative of the common garden thistle as well as the tasty artichoke. In Roman times, Pliny the Elder, a noted naturalist, described the medicinal uses of milk thistle, indicating this prickly medicine was excellent for carrying off bile.

Jean Rohrer comments:

> It has been relatively recent clinical research, especially in Germany, which has brought the use of this multifunctional plant to front row prominence in the treatment of liver toxicity. Indeed, milk thistle is considered supreme at healing chronic or acute liver damage, virtually regardless of cause, as well as protecting the liver against many toxins and pollutants…
>
> First silymarin stabilizes and strengthens liver cell walls, stopping toxins from entering. It acts by inducing formation of liver cell proteins, which are incorporated into the cell walls, making them stronger and more resistant to toxins.
>
> Second, by increasing the rate of protein synthesis, silymarin enhances regeneration of liver cells.
>
> Third, are the antioxidants and free-radical scavenging abilities of this marvelous weed. As if these impressive effects weren't sufficient, the fourth mechanism silymarin gets involved in is the enzyme and catalytic activity of the LIVER. It inhibits production of the enzymes that produce

substances damaging to the liver, while at the same time preventing the depletion of glutathione on liver cells, a substance which mediates cell metabolism…

Clinically, milk thistle causes significant reversal of symptoms of both acute and chronic liver problems from viral Hepatitis to cirrhosis (10).

During my treatment I took 400mg of milk thistle capsules 3 times daily, 30 minutes before breakfast, before lunch and before bed.

I drank 1 to 2 quarts of milk thistle tea per day.

I took 3 Hepastat 2 times per day.

I took 2 Hepata Trope 2 times per day.

Chapter Thirteen

Thymus

Enough cannot be said about Thymus. Thymus is the number one killer of the Hepatitis C virus. There are many forms: pills, liquid, natural and artificial. These all range from worthless to terrific.

One of these synthetic products is called Thymosin. It is currently being tested in several countries around the world in conjunction with Interferon. The results that have been reported are good however, Thymosin is not an item that I took, nor do I recommend it. (Refer to Appendix C: Business Wire 11/18/94).

I tried several times to purchase this product directly from the company and was denied. They did, however, advise me that I could go to Singapore. There I could purchase a large quantity of it and probably would not have any trouble bringing it back into the U.S.

The Thymus gland is a primary organ of the human immune system. It reaches maximum size during early childhood. The Thymus atrophies with age and the production of defense cells gradually declines, making humans more vulnerable to inflammatory diseases and infections.

The Thymus gland creates the T-4 "helper" white blood cells that perform their specialized job in the human body of locating invaders such as viruses, bacteria, or abnormal cells. The Thymus gland also sends out the T-8 "killer" white blood cells to find invaders and destroy them (11).

Those of us with advanced liver pathology, while feeling better after practicing my recommendations, may not completely reverse the path of the virus unless you incorporate the most aggressive and effective treatment. NatCell™ frozen Thymus extract will deliver the best possible results.

I attribute most of my successful eradication of Hepatitis C from my body as a direct result of consuming several thousand dollars of this product in eighteen months. Keep in mind that I had to pay as much as $600.00 a box to obtain the thymus from doctors. I provide this same item for less than $ 180.00. I took one frozen vial every other day. I thawed it in my hand, poured one half vial under my tongue and held it for five minutes, and repeat. If I could afford it, I would take it for the rest of my life. If Cortez had found the fountain of youth, this would have been how he felt.

You can find cheaper products, for example Thymoic Protein A, listed in *Health and Healing*, March 1997 (11). I took this product post healing. I did not notice the jolt or the feeling of well being associated with the natural form. I question whether or not it was as effective. Thymic Protein A contains only one of the seven main properties of the thymus gland.

Be warned there are some of these products that would not dissolve in water, even after an entire month.

These pass through you completely and into the toilet. If you have Hepatitis C, you need NatCell™ Thymus extract!

Thymic hormones and their down stream cell products (such as interleukins and interferons) control all phases of maturation, development, antigen commitment, proliferation and cytotoxic activity of the various T cells. Thymic hormones also stimulate non-specific phagocytic and cytotoxic cells to respond against foreign or "non-self" antigens.

Liver diseases, including chronic hepatitis and primary biliary cirrhosis, have been successfully treated by thymus extract. Results of a study using 102 patients with chronic hepatitis and primary biliary cirrhosis showed an increase in T lymphocytes, increased functional activity of mononuclear cells (increased chemotaxis and inhibition), and decreased immunoglobulin counts. All of these indicators signify an increased competence, which favors controlling the immunoinflammatory process in the liver and a normalization of the clinical manifestation of the disease leading to a favorable outcome (12).

These results are important not only for successful treatment of a very difficult disease, which frequently has an unfavorable outcome, but also for the implications for treatment of hepatitis produced by other causes. Many of the inflammatory conditions of the liver are caused by viruses, fungi, or mycobacteria (tuberculosis) (13). Cellular immunity is the chief defense against these agents. Successful treatment using thymus extracts suggests many exciting possibilities for treatment of the presently untreatable ailments of the liver using immunomodulating substances such as thymus extracts.

During my treatment I took 1 vial of NatCell thymus every other day for 18 months.

I also took 3-thymus capsules 3 times per day.

Chapter Fourteen

MEDICAL JOURNALIST REPORT OF INNOVATIVE BIOLOGICS CLINICAL APPLICATIONS OF FROZEN, LIQUID, BOVINE LIVER GROWTH FACTORS

The Pathology of Viral Hepatitis

A fairly common systemic disease, viral hepatitis is marked by hepatic cell destruction, necrosis, and autolysis; leading to anorexia, jaundice, and hepatomegaly. More than 70,000 cases of the illness are reported annually in the United States. Today, five types of viral hepatitis are recognized:

- ***Type A*** (infectious or short-incubation hepatitis). The incidence of hepatitis A is rising among homosexuals and those persons with an immunosuppression related to an infection with the human immunodeficiency virus (HIV). The ingestion of seafood from polluted waters can cause it.

- ***Type B*** (serum or long-incubation hepatitis). Also increasing among HIV-positive individuals, hepatitis B accounts for up to 10 percent of post-transfusion viral hepatitis cases in the United States. It is also transmitted by human secretions and by feces, as during intimate sexual contact and from the transfer of viruses into food prepared by infected restaurant workers.

- ***Type C*** (undetermined as to specific organism type). This disease organism is mostly acquired by blood transfusion from asymptomatic donors. Of all the hepatitis viral diseases, type C hepatitis is on the fastest rise among Americans. Hepatitis C is the most common reason for liver transplants in the U.S. today and is causing an alarming increase of primary liver cancer.

- ***Type D*** is found most frequently as a complication of acute or chronic hepatitis B, because this type D virus requires that sister organism's double-shelled surface antigen to replicate.

- ***Type E*** (formerly grouped with type C under the name *type non-A, non-B* hepatitis). It primarily occurs among people recently returned from an endemic area such as India, Africa, Asia or Central America. Of the five viral hepatitis diseases, hepatitis B and hepatitis C are most dangerous because they have a high risk of developing into liver cancer.

Defining Live Cell Liver Peptide Growth Factors

From the Department of Pathology and Laboratory Medicine at Brown University in Providence, Rhode

Island, U.S.A., three investigating pathologists, Drs. N. Fausto, A.D. Laird, and E.M. Webber, advise: "During liver regeneration quiescent hepatocytes [liver cells] undergo one or two rounds of replication and then return to a nonproliferative state. Growth factors regulate this process by providing both stimulatory and inhibitory signals for cell proliferation" (14). The idea of intrinsic hepatic growth control factors produced by animal and human liver cells has been stated in published reports, which date back as long as forty-six years ago (15,16,17,18,19). Much of this early research was conducted on rats and dogs, but currently clinical investigations among both healthy human volunteers and really sick people have taken place (20).

Comprised of the tiniest of protein molecules which biochemists and physiologists call *peptides,* these growth factors are of an exceedingly low molecular weight (30,000 Da), which yield two or more amino acids on hydrolysis. The Dalton with a symbol of D or Da, also called an *atomic mass unit,* is equivalent to 1.657 X 10 (24) gm. Peptide growth factors form by loss of water from the NH2 and COOH molecular groups of adjacent amino acids and are additionally referred to in biochemistry as di-, tri-, tetra-, etc. peptides, depending on the number of amino acids in the molecule. Thus, peptides make up the constituent parts of proteins. Examples of those several dozen peptides from the human liver and other organs which often give birth to growth factors are: hepatocyte growth factor (HGF), epidermal growth factor (EGF), transforming growth factor-beta (TGF-beta), and dozens more (20,21,22,23).

According to which of the various scientific disciplines are being queried, different names exist for peptide growth factors. Historically, for instance, cell biologists have called members of their identified growth factor-type set of molecules "growth factors"; immunologists have named their growth factor-types "interleukins," “lymphokines," or "cytokines"; while hematologists have used the growth factor-type descriptive term "colony stimulating factors" (CSF). However, the present generally delineating nomenclature of "growth factors" has been and is now, widely used throughout the world's scientific literature.

The term *growth factor* is now used consistently among almost every scientific and medical discipline because, in almost every case it reflects the context of the original discovery or isolation of any peptide. Since essentially all of these many molecules are multifunctional, it's not easy to conceive unique new names for them that would be entirely satisfactory; almost all of them are “panregulins," that is they react as universal regulators of the particular organ from which they derive. As you'll learn below, for the animal and human body, actually, peptide growth factors are physiological symbols for the transfer of signals or a kind of language of biological regulation (24,25).

Peptides often promote cell growth, but they also can inhibit it; moreover, they regulate many critical cellular functions, such as in the control of cell differentiation and other processes, which have little to do with growth itself. All peptide growth factors act in sets. To understand their actions, one must always consider the biological context in which they act.

Peptide growth factors provide an essential means for a cell to communicate with its immediate environment. They ensure that there is proper local homeostatic balance between the numerous cells that comprise a tissue or organ. Since a cell must adjust its behavior to changes in its environment, the cell needs mechanisms to provide this adaptation. Therefore, the tissue cells either singularly or collectively use sets of peptide growth factors as signaling molecules to communicate with each other and to alter their own behavior to respond appropriately to their biological context.

The most important peptide growth factors of the liver's hepatocytes have been identified as a collection of hormones called *somatomedins.* These liver hormones are peptides that produce major effects on the growth of bone and muscle. They also influence the metabolism of ingested minerals, including calcium, phosphate, carbohydrate, and lipid (fat). Somatomedin growth factors are indirectly stimulated to divide by the pituitary hormone *somatotropin* (also referred to as *growth hormone by* endocrinologists).

The peptide growth factors act by binding to functional receptors who transduct their signals and the peptides themselves may be viewed as bifunctional molecules.

The following are two main responses or actions that peptide growth factors accomplish:

(a) They possess an afferent function in that there is the conveying of information to cellular receptors, providing them with information from outside the organism's cell, tissue, or organ.

(b) They have an efferent function in that there is the inception of a latent biochemical activity of the receptor.

The Peptide Growth Factors within Liver Cells

A certain piece of geographic knowledge in nature's lore presented in the paragraph immediately below perhaps best illustrates how peptide growth factors must be considered cell-to-cell signals rather than as the equivalents of metallic parts of a machine. They offer up physiological symbols of communication within the organ systems of nearly all animal organisms. Peptides possess the unique action of serving as a significant means to convey information from one cell to another or from one organ to the next, including the brain and central nervous system, and their action in this regard is contextual.

Natural lore shows us the way peptide growth factors act to convey information inside their animal host. I ask you to visualize the reversal of host animal peptide growth factors communication in the following context: It's a fact that in two closely located islands off the coast of South Africa, a rock lobster and a large snail have reversed their predator-prey relationships. On island "Gamma" the lobster preys on the snail, finds it, attacks it, and eats its soft parts with gusto. Fifty nautical miles to the east on island "Omega," a reversal of the roles between prey and predator takes place. The same species of snail that had been eaten now preys on the same species of lobster by approaching it, extending a probing foot, burying that foot into the lobster's body, and sucking out its' gizzards (26).

What produces the reversal in predator-prey relationship? It's the host animals' peptide growth factors. Within each of the animal organisms, their growth factors alter attitude so as to become contextual; they signal differing elements of an intercellular language. To be contextual means that the whole situation, background, or environment becomes relevant to this particular animalistic prey-predator event as determined by molecular makeup of the participants' peptide growth factors.

Interleukin-6 (IL-6), one of the known peptide growth factors, regulates the protein synthesis in a human being's liver cells (hepatocytes). Also transforming growth factor-beta (TGF-beta), another set of peptide growth factors produced by normal human fibroblasts, additionally regulates the synthesis and secretion of human immunoglobulins by B-lymphocytes (25,26). Since both TGF-beta and IL-6 are also synthesized by immune cells, these molecules provide a means of communication between the immune system and its immediate neighbors. The liver is part of almost every detoxification process; therefore, the hepatocytes are often significantly involved with the metabolism of neighboring cells.

Inasmuch as the liver's natural function makes it a part of all aspects of physiological repair in the presence of body pathology, its' peptide growth factors must be critical determinants of every aspect of tissue trauma or illness response. As such, liver cell peptide growth factors have important and necessary therapeutic applications. The peptide growth factors whose functions and applications are described below by Stewart Lanson, M.D., of Scottsdale, Arizona and Howard Benedict, D.C., of New York City bring major impacts to the practice of clinical medicine and nutritional science. These peptide growth factors are involved in the repair of both soft and hard body tissues, immunosuppression, enhancement of immune cellular function, improvement of bone marrow function in numerous disease states, treatment of many proliferative diseases including the remission of cancer, the marked lowering of serum cholesterol, (29) and for the elimination of all hepatitis viral diseases, but most especially for hepatitis B and C (30).

Stuart Lanson, M.D., Treats Hepatitis C with Liver Peptides

"I use the liquid liver peptides for those of my patients who are environmentally ill with xenobiotics, allophatic hydrocarbons, pesticides, PCBs, and solvents, all stored in body fat but able to be measured in their blood in parts per billion," says Scottsdale, Arizona clinical ecologist Stuart Lanson, M.D. As medical director of the Scottsdale Ear, Nose, Throat, Allergy, and Environmental Health Center, Dr. Lanson is an allergist and holds board certification in environmental medicine. "For those patients who have problems with their detoxification systems, I employ the frozen, liquid liver extract as a standard treatment. Also I use this extract for those people suffering from the various hepatitis illnesses, most particularly for viral hepatitis C."

"For example, a woman in her early forties coming to me from a nearby Arizona city had a clear diagnosis of Hepatitis C. All of her liver enzymes were severely elevated and her symptoms included an enlarged tender liver, lethargy, poor appetite, nausea, vomiting, fever, joint pains, and jaundice," says Dr. Lanson. "I put her on multiple nutritional supplements, an elevated dosage of olive leaf extract, and NatCell™ Liver. I did this in order to have these substances work together against the virus and to strengthen my patient's liver organ. Also I treated some of her allergies with immunotherapy and preservative-free antigens," states Dr. Lanson.

"This woman has now dramatically improved. Her liver enzymes have returned to normal levels and her various symptoms have left. She reports normal amounts of energy as before she contracted hepatitis C," Dr. Lanson declares, and "my patient has now returned to work, expressed her happiness to me and basically is quite well."

"I do need to put in the limiting information that most of these hepatitis C patients do not show improvements in their viral counts. The counts continue to remain elevated even though my patients exhibit wellness and state that they feel better. The viral numbers do not seem to lower significantly," Dr. Lanson admits, and blood tests indicate that their viruses have not disappeared."

"Still, I do treat many hepatitis C patients who respond just fine to the strengthening of their liver organs by their sublingually ingesting the live cell liver treatment. This treatment overcomes their severe fatigue, impaired liver function, and elevated liver enzymes. They see noticeable symptomatic improvement! Invariably the patients' fatigue goes away, and they are able to work once again. Of course, I add other modalities besides the bovine liver growth factors, but these peptides are definitely helpful in repairing damaged liver organs. My finding is that the tiny live proteins repair a damaged liver," affirms Dr. Stuart Lanson.

Some Clinical Journal Reports of Liver Extract Enhancing Effects

Among hundreds of clinical journal research reports able to be acquired from an Internet search of Medline, here are only a few advising about the great physiological and metabolic advantages made available by liver growth factors. Research on liver growth factors was conducted both on animals and cultures in laboratories plus on sick patients receiving treatment in clinics and medical offices.

From the Department of Internal Medicine at Keio University in Tokyo, Japan, researchers report that a combined preparation of liver growth factors and flavin adenine dinucleotide (FAD) has been widely used for patients with chronic liver disease. In particular, those Japanese suffering with hepatitis C viral infections (HCV) benefited from intravenous injections of this preparation. It seems to be a potent agent to enhance the anti-viral efficacy of interferon (IFN) in patients with chronic hepatitis C (CH-C) (31).

Extracts from the weaning pig liver, although not bovine, also have acted synergistically with hepatocyte growth factors to stimulate improved function of the liver cells. The researchers did report that in the absence of added porcine growth factors, the extracts had no activity (32).

From the Third Department of Internal Medicine, National Defense Medical College in Saitama, Japan we learn about the peptide growth factor we know as Transforming Growth Factors-alpha (TGF-alpha). These particular growth factors cause biological activity when coming in contact with an extract of human exocrine pancreatic cancer associated with humoral hypercalcemia of malignancy (33).

Two mitogenic pepticles in bovine liver extracts show mitogenesis and other metabolic activity when coming in contact (in the laboratory) with basic fibroblast growth factor (FGF) (34).

Originally described as a hepatocyte peptide specific mitogen, hepatocyte growth factor (HGF) is a potent stimulator of DNA synthesis in a wide variety of cell types. It has the unique ability to transmit information that determines the spatial organization of epithelial cells in tissues as well as induce cell migration and invasion of extracellular matrix in a variety of epithelial cells. HGF is involved in physiological processes such as embryogenesis and development and in pathophysiological processes such as regeneration and carcinogenesis (35).

Investigations conducted at the University of Alabama in Birmingham, U.S.A. indicate that HGF is an important mediator of interactions for carrying on human mitogenesis, motogenesis, and morphogenesis (36).

As a mesenchymal-derived morphogen, HGF supports epithelial branching duct formation in the developing lung. **It prevents the onset or progress of hepatic fibrosis/cirrhosis and accompanying severe liver failure.** HGF may be used successfully as treatment for vascular disease, gastric ulcers, diabetes mellitus, and neuronal disease (37).

From the Department of Pathology at the University of Pittsburgh, we learn that HGF, epidermal growth factor (EGF), TGF-alpha, IL-6, tumor necrosis factor-alpha (TNF-alpha), insulin, and norepinephrine each play important roles in the sequential changes of gene expression, growth factor production, and morphologic structure (38).

The Potential Healing Benefits of Live Cell Liver Peptides

Located under the diaphragm while occupying most of the right hypochondrium and part of the epigastrium of the abdomen, the liver provides vital functions for one's body by means of its growth factors.

In preparing for our interview about his use of frozen, liquid, bovine liver peptide growth factors, Dr. Howard Benedict, a nutrition-oriented chiropractor practicing in

New York City, discussed with me the potential healing benefits of these frozen liver peptides. In summary Dr. Benedict offers the following information about the liver's numerous growth factors:

- They have vascular functions in that they cause the liver to store blood, regulate blood clotting, cleanse blood, discharge waste products into the bile, and aid the immune system by filtering the blood to remove bacteria and adding certain immune factors.

- They have secretory functions in that they aid the digestion by synthesizing and secreting bile and keeping hormones in balance.

- They have metabolic functions in that they help to manufacture new proteins; produce quick energy; regulate fat storage; control the production and excretion of cholesterol; store certain vitamins, minerals, and sugars; metabolize alcohol, carbohydrates, proteins, and fat; and proceed with detoxifying, neutralizing, and destroying xenobotic substances such as drugs, pesticides, chemicals, and pollutants.

- They are therapeutic when administered for fatty liver, hepatitis, fibrosis, cirrhosis, and damage to the liver as the result of exposure to internal and environmental toxins.

"Patients consulting me receive a functional liver assessment or test," says Dr. Benedict, “and I check their phase one and phase two metabolic liver detoxification processes. A patient's liver is challenged with caffeine or aspirin to determine its function; and if there is elevation of enzymes, tissues within the liver designed for detoxification are tested for breakdown. Liver enzyme elevation indicates such tissue breakdown. That being the case, I intervene on behalf of the patient to enhance his or her health and well being on a functional level way before there is the onset of disease."

"For those people with far advanced liver pathology, the usual orthomolecular nutritional treatment protocols such as the taking of vitamin C, alpha lipoic acid, milk thistle, curcuminoids, dandelion, green tea, and others are not enough. The more aggressive and effective treatment required is the NatCell™ Liver," Dr. Benedict advises. "Such therapy helps the patient's liver regenerate. In many situations, especially in chronic illnesses, giving someone a chance by feeding his or her ailing organ the live liver peptide growth factors, taken from a bovine source, does the job."

How to Use the Frozen, Liquid Bovine Peptide Growth Factors

Howard Benedict, D.C., conforms to the manufacturer's suggested instructions for patient and health professional use of the frozen, liquid extract. The manufacturer's product package insert tells us that the liquid extract is marketed as a food supplement only for oral use and should always be kept frozen. The insert also states:

- Peptides should be taken on an empty stomach in the morning or in the evening, either half an hour before or two hours after a meal.

- They come in a seven-cubic centimeter vial of frozen liquid that should be thawed by holding the vial in the hand.
- Shake the contents well before unscrewing the vial cap.
- Pour half of the vial's 7 cc-content (3.5 cc) under the tongue. Hold the liquid sublingually for five minutes, and then swallow it.
- Repeat this same action with the second half of liquid.
- Keep the vial closed between each step.
- According to Dr. Benedict, who adheres to the manufacturer's recommendations, use should be as a nutritional supplement at the rate of one or two vials per week.

This frozen, liquid, bovine liver peptide live cell extract may not be suitable for pregnant or nursing women and children under twelve years of age (59).

Chapter Fifteen

Reishi Mushrooms

The Reishi mushroom herb has been used for thousands of years to promote good health in the Far East.

David Law writes:

> The Reishi mushroom can increase the production of interleukin1 and 2, resulting in inhibition of tumor growth.. Studies show that Reishi can have a number of other positive effects on the body such as analgesic, anti-inflammatory, antioxidant, anti-viral (through its Interferon production), lowers blood pressure, acts as a cardiotonic (by lowering serum The Reishi Mushroom can increase the production of interleukin 1 and 2, resulting in inhibition of tumor cholesterol), expectorant, anti-tissue, liver protecting and detoxifying, protection against ionizing radiation, antibacterial, and anti-HIV activity (39).

We live in artificial environments where air is filtered, and food is processed. If we can keep our immune system functioning efficiently and strengthen our daily programs with natural immunity building supplements such as mushrooms, we can minimize the frequency and severity of illness, and recover more quickly.

To further mystify your brain into believing that the U.S. FDA has not yet graduated from kindergarten, Reishi mushrooms were used by the Chinese Chow Dynasty. This reveals that its healing properties were known by people over three thousand years ago.

The compounds found in the Reishi mushrooms have been classified as Host Defense Potentiators (HDP). These enhance the abilities of our immune system to protect itself. These disease-inhibiting compounds include Hemicellulose (AHCC), polysaccharides, polysaccharide-peptides, nucleosides, triterpeniods, complex starches, and other metabolites. In combination they strengthen the immune system, aid in neuron transmission, metabolism, hormonal balance, and the transport of nutrients and oxygen.

I strongly advocate the consumption of the natural, unadulterated and non-processed, authentic Reishi mushrooms. Purchase them in bulk, along with a seriously sharp knife for these little guys are very tough. In order to cut one into little pieces, you first must work yourself into a murderous frenzy. Make believe you're an ex-football player and commence to slay the little fungi.

I suggest only one medium size one in two quarts of water to begin. They must be simmered in a GLASS container for six hours. Then, dilute by fifty percent and drink one-half cup twice daily, between meals. Be careful of this mushroom. It can "amp" you easily. If you feel your liver swelling, drink less. It took me a while to get up to two cups a day.

You can soak the mushroom slices over night in water, then simmer for 10 minutes, strain and enjoy. Or bring water to a boil and simmer for 2-3 hours. Remember that you can only cook Reishi in a Glass Container.

These Reishi are sliced very thin and do not require the preparation I described in the chapter above.

I drink 2 cups a day.

You may also use the Reishi mushroom extract in capsule form.

Chapter Sixteen

Alpha-Lipoic Acid (ALA)

Alpha-lipoic acid is a vitamin-like antioxidant used in Europe to restore liver health and to confer protective benefits against oxidative processes involved in degenerative diseases. It is more potent than vitamins C, E and Co-Q10, and, according to Dr. Ester Packer, professor of molecular Biology at UC Berkley, may be the most important antioxidant ever discovered:

> Vitamins C, E and Glutathione work together to deactivate and prevent free radicals from causing uncontrolled damage in the body. But at this stage we run into a limiting factor regarding availability of glutathione which is an important free-radical deactivator offering protection against cataract formation, as well as immune enhancement, liver protection, cancer protection and heavy-metal detoxification.
>
> Glutathione, when taken orally like Vitamins C and E, is broken down in the stomach before it reaches the bloodstream. What does end up being absorbed can raise serum levels, but the effect inside of cells is minimal.
>
> Alpha-lipoic acid proved to be the missing link. Not only is ALA a powerful antioxidant in its own right, but it also regenerates glutathione, giving

cells a double dose of antioxidant protection. It also is easily absorbed when taken orally, and once inside cells is quickly converted to its most potent form, dihydrolipoic acid, and an even more potent free-radical neutralizer than ALA. Because both alpha-lipoic acid and dihydrolipoic acid are antioxidants, their combined actions give them greater antioxidant potency than any other natural antioxidant now known.

Scientists have also found that lipoic acid can inhibit replication of HIV-1 and other viruses through its ability to bind directly to DNA (40).

Dr. Packer and Chandan K. Sen, a researcher from Finland, have described how alpha-lipoic acid regulates aspects of the immune system, and in particular, immune cells called T-lymphocytes. They, along with other scientists, have reported how alpha-lipoic acid may help people with HIV:

"ALA inhibits growth of HIV more effectively than NAC (N-Acetyl Cysteine). Dr. Packer found in test-tube experiments, alpha-lipoic acid 'completely inhibited activation of a gene in the AIDS virus that allows it to reproduce"" (40).

Early in 1995, shortly after my diagnosis of Hepatitis C, I was consulting my brother Dwain about my will. Dwain exists in Oregon in a somewhat unusual way.

Apparently he has a radio, for it was Dwain who told me he was listening to a doctor on a talk radio program out of Seattle, who was treating Hepatitis C with 50,000 mg. injections of Vitamin C twice daily in combination with alpha-lipoic acid. ALA is a co-factor in the multi-enzyme complex that catalyzes the last stage of the process called glycolysis.

Please keep in mind, I'm not a doctor. I am a patient, who was very disappointed after spending a fortune trying to get information from doctors, and who then set out on my own to save my life.

Many, I'm sure, won't realize what a horrendous quest this was or how devastated I was because of what I discovered about our institutions.

I may write things you find offensive while others may find them quite hilarious. I don't mean to transmit any insults, my words are the way I see it. Being at the "DOOR OF DEATH" was very different than contemplating it.

Truth is stranger than fiction. This book is about truth. It's about me. I'm well and I tested negative for Hepatitis C. Whether or not my mind is regimented in a way you can take is not my concern. The remedy I put before you worked on me, and has proven to be successful on several hundred others. Healers have used much of this remedy all over the world since ancient times. A very small segment of individuals, called naturopaths, in addition to chiropractors and holistic healers have also learned things beyond what the FDA allows.

Alpha-lipoic acid occurs naturally in potatoes, sweet potatoes, carrots, yams, and red meat. I take additional alpha-lipoic acid every day, and know it has been vital in my battle and success over Hepatitis C.

I take 100mg of lipoic acid 2 times per day.

Some studies indicate taking 600mg per day can be beneficial for Hepatitis C victims.

Chapter Seventeen

Licorice Root

Licorice was brought to my attention by Candy at Pacific Coast Greens, a great health food store in Malibu. I've done some research on it, using myself as a guinea pig. I found licorice to be a wonderful herb, for it did away with all sorts of uncomfortable nuisances, e.g. high temperature, ulcers and arthritis.

Dan Mowrey states:

> Licorice root is one of the most biologically active herbs in the world...Licorice root is an effective treatment for the stomach ailments...Licorice exerts a soothing action on the muscosal surfaces of the GI tract, and is frequently used to help these tissues heal. Licorice root derivatives, glycryuhetinic acid (GLA), deglycrihyinated licorice (DGL) and carbenoxolene sodium (CS) have all been proven as among the best anti ulcer medications available... Whole licorice and its' derivatives appear to have the ability to inhibit gastric acid secretion with the advantage of being devoid of other adverse anti-cholinergic properties.
>
> Licorice root helps prevent and heal skin problems...The conditions that increase the occurrence of acne-like symptoms during certain

stages of the menstrual cycle may be affected by the consumption of licorice root.

The anti-inflammatory properties of the root have been considered responsible for its effectiveness in the treatment of numerous skin disorders, including eczema, dermatitis, impetigo and traumatized skin.

It should be mentioned that the antipyrelic (fever reducing) effects of GLA have been shown equal to those of the widely used sodium salicylate (41).

Fever reduction is important to Hepatitis C patients. My experience for several years was that I was always at about 99.8 degrees. My fever would rise after eating. It was extremely uncomfortable to live day after day, year after year, just a little bit hot.

Every time a doctor would record my slightly elevated temperature, I would ask why it was high. The usual answer was, you probably just have a bug. The licorice really helped this problem.

Licorice root is used to remove buildup of toxic metabolic substances in the body as it increases the liver's ability to filter out these wastes.

In the treatment of liver diseases (e.g. hepatitis and cirrhosis), GLA has proven extremely promising. In Chinese medicine, licorice is often used as a remedy for jaundice and is considered a great liver detoxifier.

"Experimental work has validated the usefulness of licorice in the treatment of Hepatitis, cirrhosis and related liver disorder...Licorice is a good tonic for the adrenal glands and Addison's disease" (41). This is very important for the Hepatitis C patient because you need to support your adrenal gland in many ways in order to conquer the virus.

Mowrey continues:

> Licorice appears to both mimic and potentiate the action of the adrenal-caiticosteroids, though it also differs in action from these chemicals in several important ways.
>
> Licorice components have been found to exert a positive effect on the course of several adrenal insufficiencies, even in Addison's Disease, which is characterized by near total adrenal exhaustion (41).

In later stages, the Hepatitis C patient may develop severe joint pain, which I did. This pain was compounded one hundred fold by Interferon.

Mowrey writes:

> The anti-arthritic property of GLA and of aqueous extracts of licorice have also been shown...Comparisons of licorice root to hydrocortisone are frequently made in the medical literature in England, China and countries other than the USA.
>
> In relation to the immune system, (which Hepatitis C patients must become obsessed with boosting), licorice root and its derivatives have

recently shown extremely promising results as Interferon inducers, which is especially good news for the treatment of Hepatitis C. (When was the last time your Hepatitis C doctor told you that)?

Glycyrhezic acid, at concentrations well tolerated by uninfected cells, inhibits both growth and cytopathic effect of vaccinia, as well as herpes simplex, Newcastle disease, and vesicular stomatits viruses while being ineffective on polio virus (41).

It is suggested that glycyrhezic acid interacts with virus structures (conservable proteins) producing different effects according to the viral stage affected: inactivation of free virus particles extracellularly; prevention of intercellular uncoating of infecting particles; impairment of the assembling ability of virus structural components.

"As a general cautionary measure, persons with a history of hypertension, renal failure, or the current use of cardian glycosides may wish to avoid the use of licorice root altogether" (41).

During my treatment I took 500mg 2 times per day.

I prepare the following tea every few days and drink a few cups daily.

Bring 2 quarts of water to a full boil and remove from heat. Add 3/4 cup licorice root, brew for 30 to 45 minutes and enjoy!

Chapter Eighteen

Dandelion Root

The first mention of the dandelion as medicinal was written by Arabian physicians of the tenth and eleventh centuries. Today dandelions are cultivated primarily in India as a remedy for liver disease.

The dandelion is a perennial plant found, to the dismay of many, almost everywhere. Its properties and uses include: aperient, cholague, diuretic, and tonic.

John Lust concluded:

> The dandelion has two particularly important uses; to promote the formation of bile and to remove excess water from the body in edema conditions resulting from liver problems. By acting to remove poisons from the body, it acts as a tonic and stimulant. The fresh juice is most effective, but dandelion is also prepared as a tea. An infusion of the fresh root is said to be good in gallstones, jaundice and other liver problems (42).

While I was undergoing radiation therapy for cancer, my liver count alarmed the doctor. He insisted I must be a drug addict and severe alcoholic. I begged to differ with him. On several occasions he argued with me, attempting to get me to admit something that wasn't true.

My mother, a health food fanatic of the 1950's, always told me dandelions were good for my liver. When I remembered what my mother told me about dandelions, I began drinking two quarts of dandelion tea a day. I told the Oncologist, and he insisted that there was nothing I could take that would lower my liver count. That I should just stop drinking and using drugs.

After one month of drinking two quarts of dandelion tea a day, my ALT count dropped fifty points. Since then, I've been taking dandelion root everyday.

During my treatment I took 500mg of dandelion root 3 times per day.

I made tea from the Dandelion Root and drank about 1 quart every evening.

Bring two quarts of distilled water to a full boil. Pour in 1 cup dandelion root. Simmer for 15 minutes, remove from heat and let brew for 1 hour.

Strain and enjoy.

I keep a large supply in the refrigerator and drink as iced tea.

Chapter Nineteen

Cats Claws
(Uncaria Tamentosa)

Cats Claws is an herb that grows in the rain forest of the Peruvian Amazon. Native Peruvian Indians have used it for centuries, dating back to the ancient Incas. The inner bark contains unique active constituents to help support the body's natural defenses.

Cats Claws is currently the subject of extensive scientific research and is used worldwide as a nutritional supplement.

I discovered Cats Claw on the Internet while desperately seeking a cure for hepatocellular carcinoma. The immediate suggestion of dying from this disease was related to me by the blood donor bank technician, who informed me of my Hepatitis C infection. He suggested that my final demise would be from that wonderful form of cancer, since there was no possible way to alter the death path of Hepatitis C. Mickey Mantle, Alan Ginsburg and many other famous people have died from hepatocellular carcinoma, as a complication of Hepatitis C.

Unknown to most Americans, Cats Claw is sold over the counter in most South American countries and labeled as a cancer cure. It has terrific anti-viral qualities as well and should not be overlooked in your quest for life.

Six Oxindole Alkaloids have been isolated from the inner bark. These Oxindole Alkaloids have been proven to provide a general boost to the immune system and have a profound effect on the ability of white blood cells to engulf and digest harmful microorganisms and foreign matter. Other Alkaloids and phytochemicals present in Cats Claw have been shown to provide natural support against many viruses.

Besides containing Oxindole Alkaloids, Peruvian and Italian researchers have discovered a wealth of other beneficial phytochemicals inherent in the herb, including proanthacyanidens, polyphenols, triterpines and plant sterols beta- stitosterol, stigmasterol and campesterol. The presence of these additional compounds might further explain the anti-oxidant, anti-microbial, anti-tumor and anti-inflammatory properties attributed to this herb. This herb is a powerful cellular reconstitutor.

In the words of Dr. Brent Davis, "Uncaria Tomentosa (Cats Claw) is a world class herb which has the power to arrest and reverse deep seated pathology, allowing a more rapid return to health in the context of consistent A. K. therapies'" (43).

During my treatment I made tea from the inner bark.

Bring 2 quarts water to a boil

Add 1 cup shredded bark

Simmer for 15 minutes then let brew for 1 hour.

Strain and enjoy!

I also took 250mg capsules 2 times per day.

Chapter Twenty

Aloe Vera

Dr. John Finnegan, N. D. found:

Mucopolysaccharides are made in the human body and perform many key functions in our health, including growth and immune system functioning. Unfortunately, after puberty we cease manufacturing these and must obtain them from outside sources. Mucopolysaccharides are found in large amounts in fresh aloe vera and in properly prepared aloe vera juices. Following are a few of the vital functions that mucopolysaccharides have been found to perform.

- They become incorporated into the cellular membrane and make the cell more resistant to the viruses and pathogenic bacteria.
- They improve overall cellular metabolism and functioning.
- They have anti-inflammatory properties.
- They provide critical lubrication of joints; helping to prevent arthritis and to heal it once it has developed.
- They aid in the absorption of water, minerals and nutrients in the GI track.

- They improve macrophage (white blood cell) activity making them up to ten times more effective in engulfing foreign matter.
- They enhance the macrophage's effectiveness in modulating the entire immune system.
- They enhance the macrophage's effectiveness to stimulate and direct the production and release of antibodies (increasing the body's own production of interferon, interleukins and more).
- They increase the number of antibody forming T-cells in the spleen as well as increase the number and activity of killer T-cell and monocyte activity.
- They are responsible for aloe's special penetration properties.
- In conjunction with their cellular detoxification support and immune enhancement, they improve allergic reactions.
- They stimulate bone marrow activity.
- They stimulate the fibroblasts to release collagen and elastin to make new tissue (inside and out).
- These mucopolysaccharides in aloe vera enhance the functioning of the entire immune, repair, detoxification, digestive and elimination systems of the body (44).

Dr. John Finnegan prescribed aloe vera for me and at the time I had no idea that it was anything more than an expensive cactus juice. After taking it for two days, the diarrhea I'd had most of the time since my four blood transfusions was gone. There was a true feeling of reversal from sicker and sicker to a leveling off and a healing taking place. Of course Dr. John Finnegan prescribed several things in the first few months, only a few of which I could afford. Aloe Vera was one item I purchased by the case from him. He has had great successes in using aloe with his Hepatitis clients. Properly prepared Aloe Vera is a must in the quest against Hepatitis C. In chronic Hepatitis C cases there is suffering from severe joint pain. Aloe Vera helped eliminate this pain for me better than anything else I've tried. Its' cost can drive you to the poor house, but at least the physical suffering on the way isn't as bad. Wouldn't it be great if you were one of those fortunate enough to have insurance and they would pay for at least a portion of this product. It's better than most things you'll ever buy in a bottle.

Immune Enhancing Effects of Aloe

by John Pittman, M.D.

Beta- Glucomannans are a class of very long chain sugars derived from plants, which have been shown in laboratory and clinical studies to have a wide variety if immune stimulating and protective effects within the body. In studying the different sources of this polymer, it has been discovered that the aloe barbadensis plant contains the greatest concentration of acetylated polymannans, which is also the most active form of mannans. These long-chain complex polysaccharides are often called Beta-Glucomannans, Mucopolysaccharides or Acemannan. These aloe polysaccharides have been shown to have many effects in the body, mostly impacting the gastrointestinal and immune systems, which are intricately related. Before elaborating on their beneficial effects, it is appropriate to discuss the type of pathology often present in individuals experiencing immune system depression.

The most striking commonality found in individuals suffering with immune depressive conditions (Epstein-Bar virus, Chronic Fatigue Syndrome, systemic candidiasis, HIV infection and others) is their high incidence of digestive dysfunction and maldigestion. This has several effects that contribute to stress on the immune system and therefore its weakening.

Maldigestion means that the consumed food is not properly broken down into the elemental building blocks needed for the body to rebuild itself and to generate energy for metabolism. This results in a type of starvation at the cellular level, with all tissue suffering malnourishment and therefore decreased effectiveness of all internal chemical processes.

These processes include breakdown and transport of toxins out of the cell, movement of nutrients into the cell, and energy production for cell functioning. This affects all the cells in the body, including those of the immune system such as white blood cells, (macrophages, and lymphocytes) and red blood sells which carry oxygen throughout our bodies. Not only do we lack enough fuel but we're low on oxygen too.

However, it is not this cellular starvation alone that causes the immune depression. Maldigestion also results in pathologic reactions. First, these remnants become irritants and cause inflammation of the mucosal wall of the intestines. Many powerful enzymes and damaging chemicals are released, injuring the intestinal wall causing increased intestinal mucosal permeability. The foreign proteins of the digested food can leak across the mucosa into the lymphatic channels of the intestinal wall and from there, gain access to the circulatory system. Here, these absorbed proteins are recognized as foreign and are attacked by the cells of the immune system. Antibodies bind to the protein and then call in the macrophages and monocytes. T-cells arrive later, releasing enzymes and using oxygen to drive the metabolic breakdown of the foreign protein. The total result is that the immune system is constantly turned on and draining down like a battery. As these allergic reactions to food breakdown products continue, the cells of the Immune system wear out faster, run out of fuel and aren't reproduced in sufficient numbers.

In addition to this chronic hyperimmune state, undigested food remnants provide fuel for overgrowth of fermentative fungal organisms such as Candida albicans as well as several types of parasites. Overgrowth of Candida in the intestines has significant effects throughout the body due to the absorption of toxic by-products of its metabolism. This can result in worsening of food allergies, hypoglycemia, digestive disturbances, excessive mucus, bloating, flatulence, skin rashes and extreme fatigue. This chronic infection further drains the immune system and complicates the picture.

Further damage is inflicted on all cell membranes from the effects of the generalized inflammation occurring as a result of maldigestion. These metabolic reactions utilize large amounts of oxygen and produce oxidative free radicals as waste by-products. The negatively charged oxygen molecules are desperately trying to balance their electrical charge and immediately begin to chop holes into cell membranes as they grab positive charges. The result here is further damage to the intestinal mucosa and a worsening of the increased permeability.

All these processes work together in a vicious sequence of events leading to progressive weakening of the immune system. It is clear that many mechanisms are at play in orchestrating these processes. Without definitive therapy directed at each component of the immune system pathology, this is a downward spiral to death. Fortunately, a thorough multidimensional treatment protocol addressing each component has been shown to reverse these processes. Aloe vera has been shown to have properties addressing all these issues and appears to play a key role on many different levels in boosting all immune functioning.

At the intestinal level, the aloe polysaccharides have been shown to act as potent anti-inflammatory agents, neutralizing many of the enzymes responsible for damaging the mucosal wall and, in effect, quenching the fire. They do this anti-inflammatory action while at the same time boosting the immune system functioning. This results in decreased leakiness of the intestinal wall and less absorption of allergic stimulating foreign protein as well as enhancing the repair of the tissue. Research has also demonstrated their direct viricidal, bactericidal, and fungicidal properties, which can help control candida overgrowth so the normal gastrointestinal bacterial flora can be restored. It has also been found that these polysaccharides stimulate intestinal motility, improving the elimination process to move allergenic proteins from the small intestine into the colon. All these processes help to normalize gastrointestinal wall structure and function and therefore stop the viscous cycle of immune system damage.

In addition to restoring gastrointestinal and elimination functioning, these large glucomannan polysaccharides also have direct effects on the cells of the immune system.

They have been shown to increase the number of and activate the intensity of macrophages, monocytes, and T-cells as well as increasing the number of antibody forming B-cells in the spleen. Enhancing macrophage activity increases the effectiveness of the entire immune and repair system of the body as it is responsible for so many functions, including immune modualtion.

These polysaccharides have been shown in laboratory studies to act as a bridge between foreign proteins (such as virus particles) and the macrophage, facilitating phagocytosis ingestion of the protein by the macrophage. Activating the receptor sites of the macrophages is a key to the overall boosting of cell-mediated immunity, which is deficient in HIV infection and other immune disorders. These aloe polysaccharides also protect the bone marrow from damage by toxic chemicals and drugs.

These various effects, while seemingly wide spread and unrelated, are in fact due to one simple process at the cell membrane level. Acemannan (the name often used for aloe beta-glucomannans, acetylated polymannans and mucopolysaccharides) is a long chain sugar that interjects itself into all cell membranes. This results in an increase in the fluidity and permeability of the membranes allowing toxins to flow out of the cell more easily and nutrients to enter the cell. This results in improved cellular metabolism throughout the body and an overall boost in energy production. The vicious cycle of maldigestion and cellular starvation is finally broken as the Acemannan normalizes absorption of nutrients and increases tolerance for allergenic foods (from detoxification). The immune system is now stronger, under control, and better prepared for any new threat.

As humans living in the late twentieth century, our body's metabolic and detoxification systems are under ever increasing stress from foreign chemicals, nutrient depleted foods, and immune damaging infectious agents.

In order to control and prevent the inevitable progression of the immune system destruction that these stresses cause, therapy must be multifactorial involving all levels of health, diet and lifestyle. These different areas consist of destruction of pathogenic organisms, metabolic detoxification, intestinal cleansing, increasing cellular metabolism, antioxidant agents to combat free radicals, and direct stimulation of immune system cells. Aloe vera's Acemannan, the active ingredient in cold-processed, whole leaf aloe has been demonstrated in laboratory testing and clinical use to be effective on all levels of this therapeutic program (45).

The Secret Promise of Aloe Vera

by Dr. Jeri L. Heyman, Ph.D.

I am a developmental psychologist who has focused on psychological and emotional development for most of my life and career. By becoming aware of the latest research on Aloe Vera I have become inspired to examine healthy physical development more closely in addition to the biochemical contribution to overall optimal health and balance. I found the Aloe Vera plant to be the most fascinating and miraculous plant on the planet. I have spent the last five years investigating Aloe Vera, and it keeps getting more interesting all the time. As you begin to look at the information on Aloe, you may find conflicting information. Please be aware that there is still a great deal of misinformation and misunderstandings about Aloe Vera and Aloe Vera products. It is very hard to believe that all the scientific research on the properties of fresh Aloe Vera could possibly be real - but they are.

The research raised many questions for me. How could something be so profoundly and fundamentally effective for so many areas of health and have only good side effects? Why (if this research is real and Aloe has been around for so long) haven't we heard more about experiences of these miraculous effects? What I found is that the research on fresh Aloe Vera is real and the research on the constituents in fresh Aloe is real. However, most Aloe Vera products available in the marketplace, although they can have some benefits, are not demonstrating the promises documented by the research. Thus, Aloe Vera's true potential has remained a secret.

The Effectiveness of Aloe Vera - Fundamental and Profound.

The Immune System:

Scientific research has demonstrated so many healthful properties of Aloe that one's immediate response has to be, "this can't be real". Aloe Vera enhances the body's own health and healing in so many ways that I wouldn't even have dreamed to pray for them all. Certainly I couldn't have imagined that they would be found all in one plant, in a natural form and with only good side effects.

It was discovered that fresh Aloe Vera contains over 250 constituents including the full range of all sizes of polysaccharides (complex sugar chains that feed the cells). The largest long-chain polysaccharides have an intricate, multifacted, multifunctional biological design and are manufactured by the body only until puberty. After puberty we must get these health and growth producing polysaccharides from outside sources. Aloe Vera has been found to be the most concentrated plant source of these largest known and most profound health supporting polysaccharides - the Beta-Glucomannans (also known as Mucopolysaccharides, Acemannan, Acetylated Polymannose).

Research by a pharmaceutical company, Carrington Laboratories, has documented some of the astounding properties of the various sizes of Aloe Vera long-chain sugars. As reported by Dr. Ivan Danhof, they discovered that the smaller-chained polysaccharides have properties that help in balancing blood sugar levels. Although this is still being studied, there is evidence that they improve insulin receptor cells, with importance for both Type I and Type II diabetes (not to mention balancing sugar cravings). The research has also demonstrated some anti-inflammatory properties of these smaller polysaccharides as they mimic the action of steroids. The medium size polysaccharides have been found to be potent antioxidants. The larger chains have demonstrated direct antibacterial properties (staph, strep, E coli...), direct antiviral properties (herpes, influenza, HIV) and the stimulation body's own tissue regeneration processes (by fitting receptor sites of fibroblasts stimulating them to produce collagen and other factors needed to make new tissue).

The largest longest-chained polysaccharides, the Beta-Glucomannans (Mucopolysaccharides), have received the most attention and Carrington has patented the Beta 1,4 Glucomannan, as "Acemannan". They documented astounding immune enhancing and tissue production properties of this Aloe polysaccharide. They actually showed that when the Acemannan meets the receptor sites of macrophages it stimulates the macrophage into action and can increase its affectivity ten fold. The macrophages are the main immune system cells. They are the white blood cells that engulf foreign matter throughout the body, release growth factor to stimulate tissue generation, modulate the inflammation processes and more. They command the other immune cells to release their antibodies- how much, when and where needed.

Carrington's research showed that when the macrophage is stimulated it does increase the production and release of interferon and the interleukins when needed. This fascinates me because here is a natural way that actually helps the body's own mechanisms to increase antibody production as well as increase the effectiveness of getting to where its needed. The body was designed with all the mechanisms to heal itself. Here there is a way to enhance the body's own systems for healing! The macrophages are also responsible for orchestrating and modulating all the other immune cells and the entire immune system's functioning. They command the immune cell army, signaling where to go, when and how hard to attack and when to cease-fire.

So the question of how can one polysaccharide be so great for so many things is partly answered here because the macrophage does so many profound things and the beta-glucomannan is making it 10 times more effective. So, when the literature on Aloe Vera is talking about direct immune enhancement they are referring to this body of research on polysaccharides by Carrington Laboratories.

Supporting Fundamental Health by

"Re-Naturing" the Cells.

Macrophage stimulation and direct immune system support is just part of the story of how Aloe can have such a broad range of health benefits. Aloe Vera is known to be the most penetrating and absorbing of substances. It moves through cells and tissues like no other substance on earth. Research has shown that fresh Aloe will absorb through to all seven layers of skin. Understanding this action has profound implications understanding the effects of Aloe for cellular health. The Aloe, led by the large polysaccharide, is of a unique size and shape as to be able to penetrate cell walls dramatically. Sometimes the polysaccharides can become part of the cell membrane fortifying the cell wall. Sometimes the Aloe moves into a cell, bringing all its nutrients and co-factors and also cleanses the cells by taking toxins out. The Aloe feeds, nourishes, fortifies and cleanses the cell, improving cellular metabolism and the cell's optimal functioning. I call this "Re-Naturing" the cell because it can feed the cell in such a way as to make it function as it was originally designed by Nature. The health benefits of this one property of fresh Aloe are mind-boggling. Here is a plant that can improve the health of the cells throughout the body. When the cells are healthy and functioning as they should, all the tissues, glands, organs and systems of the body are also getting "Re-Natured".

A Myriad of Nutrients and Co-Factors supporting overall Healthy Functioning.

Dr. Robert Davis has done a great deal of research on fresh Aloe Vera, the properties of its many nutrients and how the Aloe polysaccharides work. Research has found that in addition to the full range of sizes of polysaccharides, fresh Aloe contains over 250 other constituents including: vitamins (the only plant source of vitamin B12); minerals; amino acids; essential fatty acids; a natural form of salicylic acid and plant sterols (with antiseptic, anti-inflammatory and analgesic properties); enzymes (including two that the body needs of which Aloe is the only plant source); glycoproteins; and more. These constituents have properties of their own as well as serve as co-factors and support for many of the body's biochemical processes. Dr. Davis' research, as explained below, shows that all the nutrients in Aloe Vera are crucial to the Aloe polysaccharides' effectiveness and biological availability throughout the body.

Isolated Nutrients Extracted by Science vs. the Original Designs Created by Nature.

Carrington Laboratories isolated and patented Acemannan. They continued their research with orally ingested capsules of Acemannan, isolated from freeze dried Aloe. The clinical results must not have given them the results they expected as they switched to the study of injectible Acemannan for which they have FDA approval for study with animals and humans. What does this tell us? I can't imagine that a pharmaceutical company would rather patent an injectible over a capsule. It certainly made me wonder that maybe the research findings only are experienced if the polysaccharides are injected right into where they are needed.

Is this why we haven't heard of these miraculous immune enhancing effects? Is it because the digestive system destroys the polysaccharides? Is it because the polysaccharides can't get through to the lymph system?

It is Dr. Davis' explanation of his Conductor/Orchestra Theory that most helped me begin to understand Aloe's Secret Promise. Dr. Davis describes how the entire Aloe molecule, with the polysaccharides laced in perfect balance with the other myriad of constituents within a base of water, is what is necessary for the Aloe polysaccharides to be available throughout the body and to effectively demonstrate the research on the polysaccharides. The polysaccharide acts as the conductor of the orchestra of all other nutrients. It is the entire "orchestra" that is responsible for the benefits of Aloe "being heard" throughout the body.

As I understand it, the Aloe molecule is balanced with the polysaccharide on one end and the other constituents as the "orchestra" on the other end, making it slightly charged on each end. In this form the Aloe moves through tissue and throughout the body with the biological design that has a biological wisdom and intercellular communication properties. The Aloe works its way to special receptor sites in the digestive tract that ingests the Aloe led by the largest polysaccharides and brings it in "whole" into the lymph system where it is then available to move throughout the body and "know" where to go. Our immune cells send out "chemotaxic" signals when "in need of assistance" that other immune cells as well as the whole Aloe are drawn to.

Thus, it is in its "whole" form that the aloe polysaccharides are most biologically active and biologically available to the cells of the body. The isolated polysaccharide lacks the biological wisdom and ability to "move" throughout the body to the cells in need. Thus, the properties of polysaccharides that are not in their original design within the Aloe will only "work" when they happen to "hit on" particular cells.

It is of critical importance that the Aloe not only contain the full range of sizes of polysaccharides but that they also need to be in their originally designed form and balance. Thus, the full promise of Aloe Vera with all the properties that the research has documented will only be fully demonstrated if the Aloe Vera is intact.

Why Aloe Vera's True Promise has Been Hidden:

So, again, I ask myself - if this research is real then why aren't we hearing more about these miraculous effects of drinking Aloe Vera? And why are the Aloe Vera gels on the market just O.K. and not the miraculous tissue regenerating gel that the research suggests?

Processing, Processing, Processing! It dawned on me when I used two different Aloe Juice products that were labeled the exact same way - whole leaf, cold processed, aloin removed - but they tasted different (aloin) and were not equally effective. As my Aloe investigation and search for a "good" Aloe continued I learned it is important to read labels very carefully - what they say and do not say are both important.

It makes sense that if the fresh, whole Aloe "works" then we need an Aloe that is as close to fresh as possible.

Processed Aloe Vera vs. its Original Biological Design.

Although the research is real, the effectiveness of any given aloe product will depend on what "is in" and what "is not in" a given product. Demonstration of the scientific research's promises will depend on having the full range of sizes of polysaccharides in the form they need to be to work best in the body. Thus, any processing of the Aloe (to stabilize and purify) needs to capture and protect all the constituents as well as maintain their original design and balance. Beware of an Aloe product that does not guarantee, in writing, that no heat is ever applied from field to bottle. Beware of concentrated or dried Aloes. The processing can damage constituents as well as their not being in the original proportions and design. Aloin is a bitter substance found in Aloe that has unwanted, irritating, laxative properties and is responsible for the contraindications for daily use. Be sure your Aloe juice has the aloin removed to less than 10 ppm (laxation occurs at around 2ppm).

Heat and Biological Activity.

Heat can be the most damaging to the important Aloe nutrients. Heat can break down the links between the sugars. When this happens, the long chain sugars no longer have the same size and shape of the polysaccharides that fit the receptor sites of key immune cells and tissue producing cells, nor do they have the other properties that the research has documented.

Heat also breaks down the structure of the enzymes and can also damage amino acids and all the other nutrients. Cells are designed with a biological structure that breaks down with heat above body temperature. As I understand it, the body's fever that is produced when all else is failing, helps to kill cells, but unlike other aspects of the immune system, heat does not discriminate between our own cells and foreign cells. Thus, it seems logical that temperatures of 100F- 110F are designed to kill the biological activity (life) of cells in our own bodies. I used to think a fever was a side effect of the body not having enough energy to effectively fight off an illness. But that doesn't make sense to me anymore. If the body has no energy for maintaining the homeostasis (balance) of temperature, it is more likely that the body's temperature would drop. When the immune system is being overtaxed and failing it fires up and uses heat to help to break down and destroy the biological structure for life and growth.

This focus on fever highlights the importance of "biological temperatures". When the Aloe Vera (or any food) is heated, intricate biological structures are destroyed along with their biological benefits. Additionally, for Aloe Vera, heat not only destroys the important polysaccharides, enzymes and more but also destroys the balance of the entire Aloe molecule and thus its biological availability and effectiveness throughout the body.

Our Bodies are Perfectly Designed.

Our body is designed in perfect balance to take in, absorb and eliminate nutrients and process and eliminate foreign and toxic matter, fight off ills, repair tissue and grow. If given the proper tools, the body is designed to be healthy and strong. The best thing we could do for our bodies is to feed it the nutrients it needs, limit the toxins taken in, not to overtax any one system and to protect the balance of all the systems. So look at what we are doing: we are not eating enough raw organic foods that contain the nutrients we need in the form we need them; we are eating mostly cooked foods which changes the nutrients to forms that not only do not feed the body but can burden the body; by age five the toxins in our environment have overtaxed all the systems of our bodies; we take medicines that put the digestive system out of balance and do nothing to restore that balance and healthy functioning, thus starting a domino effect of problems that eventually overtax the entire immune system's functioning.

All of our body's "ills" can be traced to the body's own systems not working well. Medicine is designed to be crisis intervention (and I am grateful for this) not nutritional health support. We need to learn ways to work with our bodies to support the perfectly designed systems we have. When we treat symptoms of illness, we can be interfering with our natural "wellness" processes. Often we are counteracting the body's own wisdom and mechanisms for health. Is diarrhea a sign of illness? Yes and No. Yes, it is a sign that the body is overloaded with waste that needs to be flushed. But no, it is a sign of wellness in that it is flushing the waste from successful immune warfare. Diarrhea is not an illness, per se. It is a result of the body's fighting an "illness" from harmful microorganisms. What an ingenious wellness system: when the fluids from the fight (mucous) build up, the body takes water and mucous from the system and "flushes" the toxins out.

Enough on that system, let's move on. Think about the mucous produced with allergies and viruses. It is a waste product that needs to be eliminated. We need to help the body get rid of the mucous, not stop it from coming out. When we stop the mucous elimination process, what happens to the toxic waste? We don't need things to dry up the mucous, but we could use a "flush button" that would get rid of it in 5 minutes! I wish all the resources for medical science were actually focused on wellness!

Our environment and the foods we eat are overtaxing our body's ability to eliminate toxins. Traditional approaches to health care and medicine not only can destroy the digestive system but also overtax the elimination system, especially the liver. When we stop the symptoms of an illness, we are clogging up the body's immune and elimination systems' natural processes. We can be stopping the body's natural wellness process trying to rid the body of toxic waste. When we do this, we end up overloading the other systems of elimination, especially the kidneys and liver even more.

Aloe Vera - The Herbal Answer to Today's Health Crisis.

Aloe Vera is the best herbal answer I can imagine to support the health and healing mechanisms of the body because "IT" doesn't heal, rather, it FEEDS THE BODY'S OWN SYSTEMS to function optimally and be healthy. It does this, in part, by going into the cells and "Re-Natures" them to function optimally, as they were originally designed. Thus is a fundamental tool to feed life to the cells, tissues, glands, organs, and systems of the body to support optimal health, balance and functioning. In addition Aloe Vera has been shown to have many specific properties that profoundly enhance the functioning of body's own immune/repair systems for health and healing to be up to ten times more effective, thus healing can be ten times faster. Aloe Vera is a remarkable plant. I urge everyone to examine this for him or her self. To understand that nutrients designed by nature were designed to feed our body perfectly is to understand the importance of feeding the body the fuel it needs to function optimally, as it was originally designed.

The Promise in the Aloe Vera plant has opened my eyes to how we need to look to Nature's original designs for life - to feed life, development and health. It is as though GOD put the Aloe Vera plant here not only as a gift for health but also as a metaphor for the miracles possible if we "Trust the Divine Design".

During my treatment I drank 4oz. of properly prepared Aloe Vera 2 - 4 times per day, usually more. By properly prepared I mean raw (unheated), organic, whole leaf and never concentrated or diluted aloe with all the aloin (laxative properties) removed.

It is fortunate that the Aloe Vera, recommended by Dr. Finnegan, happened to be a unique aloe product (enhanced with fantastic immune herbs) that is processed in a special way. You just can't get any aloe product. The processing will determine what is "in" and "what's not in" the aloe and will determine the results. Once again it is difficult to know the truth about products. So make sure your aloe company guarantees - in writing - that heat is never applied from field to bottle and that it never experiences temperatures above 90F at any time during processing, that it has never been concentrated or diluted, that the whole leaf is being used (more potent) and that the aloin (which can irritate the bowel) is completely removed to 1ppm or less without any damaging processing. Remember, if it's not written on the bottle you can't assume anything.

Chapter Twenty-One

Vitamin C

Hans Larsen states:

> Vitamin C was first isolated in 1928 by the Hungarian biochemist and Nobel Prize winner Dr. Syent-Gyorgijc. Vitamin C plays an important role as a component of enzymes involved in the synthesis of collagen and carnitine.
>
> Vitamin C intake markedly reduces the severity of a cold; it also effectively prevents secondary viral and bacterial complications. Vitamin C works by stimulating the immune system and protecting against damage by the free radicals released by the body in its fight against the infection (46).

Drs. Pauling and Cameron pioneered the use of large doses of Vitamin C (more than 10 grams a day) in the treatment of cancer patients. From their experiments at the Vale of Leven Hospital in Scotland, they concluded that terminal cancer patients who received large daily doses of Vitamin C, along with the regular treatment, lived much longer than patients who did not receive Vitamin C. These patients also had less pain, and in general, a much-improved quality of life.

Larsen continues:

> Vitamin C is truly a wonder nutrient and there is no doubt that many of the serious degenerative diseases plaguing the civilized world today can be prevented or even reversed through an adequate intake of this essential vitamin.
>
> A scientific advising panel to the US government recently recommended that all healthy adults increase their Vitamin C intake to 250-1000 mg a day.
>
> A daily intake of 250-1000 mg of Vitamin C may be adequate for preventive purposes, but far larger quantities are required in halting or reversing cancer and heart disease and Hepatitis C.
>
> Although there has been some concern that people suffering from hemochromatosis (a tendency to iron overload) may be sensitive to high doses of Vitamin C, most researchers agree that Vitamin C is entirely safe in daily quantities of 10 grams or more. An adequate intake of Vitamin C is surely the best and most cost efficient health insurance available today (46).

The official Recommended Daily Allowance (RDA) is sixty mg. per day. How much do we need? To answer this question it is crucial to realize that the RDA is not, in any way, based on what is required for optimum health. The RDA is simply the amount required to avoid scurvy, the most obvious deficiency disease. Actually the RDA is based on the Vitamin C content of the average diet. The logic goes somewhat like this: The average "healthy" North American diet provides about 60 mg. per day of Vitamin C, so since scurvy is virtually unknown in the USA today, 60 mg. per day must be adequate. So much for Science.

High-potency Vitamin C produces dramatic healing in many Hepatitis C patients. I used C Aspa Scorb by Progressive Laboratories, Inc. It comes in powder form and the dose recommended is one teaspoon, three times a day or approximately fourteen thousand (14,000) mg. This product also contains Selenium 270 mg.

Research papers have reported that RNA viruses, including Hepatitis C, encode selenium-dependent glutathione peroxide genes. Research indicates that selenium may act as a "birth control pill" for the virus.

You mix a teaspoon full in a small amount of distilled water or juice.

When I first employed Dr. D for my liver problem, his first diagnosis was hemochromatosis. This was, according to him, an inherited disease. He asked if any of my relatives had had the disease? Most of my relatives were dead from cancer, so I didn't know.

I experienced a horrendous iron overload in my liver. Chronic Hepatitis C does cause iron overload mostly in male patients, and there are several known adverse effects. I'm sure a lot of unknown problems result from iron overload. That is why Dr. D prescribed phlebotomies or bloodletting, to leach the iron from my liver. My bloodletting led to the blood bank discovering my Hepatitis C.

Drinking distilled water helps leach out iron and other toxic overloads from the liver. All chronic Hepatitis C patients should drink distilled water during the night.

As long as we're on the topic of iron retention, it is important for Hepatitis C patients to avoid all iron supplements. Carefully read the ingredients in supplements because iron is added needlessly in all sorts of pills and other types of supplements such as super-foods and in particular supplements designed for women. If you have Hepatitis C and don't know if you're retaining iron in your liver, get tested. A simple blood test will reveal your iron binding content. If you have a liver biopsy, be sure to remind your doctor to have an iron test done at the same time. Not all doctors know or remember to do this. In my case they did do it, but they lost it. I wasn't about to visit Dr. "Pocahontas" a second time.

For Vitamin C, I consumed at least two lemons everyday. They should be fresh and organic. Use them in tea, to marinate meat, in stir-fry and to make lemonade, lemon honey and distilled water. Put a slice of lemon in your glass of water, it makes water exciting. There are live enzymes and bioflavonoids in fresh squeezed fruit that just isn't in pills, powder or processed supplements. Also, lemons are a good source of the mineral magnesium, which helps maintain the mineral balance in the body.

Maud Grieve, a modern herbalist said, "It is probable that the lemon is the most valuable of all fruit for preserving health" (47).

During my treatment I took 7000mg of vitamin C 2 times per day for three months.

I then cut down to 2000mg 2 times per day.

Vitamin C can leach calcium out of your bones, so I suggest taking a calcium supplement in addition to the Vitamin C.

Chapter Twenty-Two

Alfalfa (Medicago Sativa)

For centuries, alfalfa has been referred to as the father of all foods.

Alfalfa was first cultivated in Persia. In five hundred BC it was then taken to Greece. Alfalfa spread until one day in 1854, it arrived in San Francisco, the American incubator of all good herbs.

Alfalfa has a very unique and distinctive quality that sets it apart from most other plants. The root system of the Alfalfa plant reaches thirty feet deep into the soil. This allows the plant to access a large quantity of un-depleted nutrients, salts, and necessary elements, while most other plants simply don't have this advantage. The leaves of Alfalfa contain the eight essential amino acids and ten "non-essential" amino acids. (Refer to Appendix D for a list of its ingredients).

Alfalfa is useful in the treatment of arthritis, urinary tract, kidney and bladder infections, as well as prostate disorders. Alfalfa alkalizes and detoxifies the body, especially the liver.

Studies have shown that Alfalfa has inhibited the growth of viruses such as herpes simplex. L-canaverine, a non-protein amino acid, found in Alfalfa leaves and roots, has been shown in animal studies to have anti-viral properties and be effective in controlling leukemia and cancer cells.

During my treatment I took 1 gram of Alfalfa 2 times per day.

Chapter Twenty-Three

Nicotinamide Adenine Dinucleotide (NADH)

NADH is an incredible supplement, especially for those of you who have undergone the unfortunate use of Interferon. One of Interferon's best-known side effects is to interfere with the neurotransmissions in the brain stem. In this area of the brain there are approximately fifteen billion brain cells. The messages that come in through your five senses and other important bodily functions are transmitted between these cells by neurotransmitters.

"NADH is required for synthesis of neurotransmitters which explains its effects on maintaining healthy mind and mental functions. NADH is the co-enzymatic form of vitamin B-3. NADH is involved in production of energy in all cells" (48).

In my case, Interferon so devastated these transmissions that I could not draw a simple line between numbers on a test given to me by a state appointed neurologist / psychiatrist. He explained to me that the use of Interferon has resulted in symptoms very similar to those of the Gulf War Syndrome.

During and ever since my exposure to that toxic garbage, my ability to cut a straight line with my skill saw has been eradicated. My once perfected ability as a master carpenter has been erased forever.

I strongly recommend NADH for all who suffer from Hepatitis C. Try it and you'll see why. It is well worth the buck a pill.

During my treatment I took 2.5mg of NADH every morning.

Chapter Twenty-Four

Cleanliness and Albumin

Cleanliness is a key factor in the control and prevention of all disease.

In Exodus 15:26 we find:

> If thou wilt diligently hearken to the voice of the Lord thy God, and wilt do that which is right in his sight, and wilt give ear to his commandments, and keep all his statutes, I will put none of these diseases upon thee, which I have brought upon the Egyptians: for I am the Lord that healeth thee (49).

Numbers Chapter 19:

> And the Lord spoke unto Moses and unto Aaron saying… You can look it up and read it for yourself. God prescribed detailed methods for using water, various herbs and drying time to cleanse the body properly under several different circumstances: in dealing with the dead, for the prevention of spreading disease, bacteria, viruses and also for the washing of cloths.

McMillan recounts:

In the early 1840's a young doctor named Ignay Semmelweis was given charge over one of the obstetrical wards. He observed that those women who were examined became sick and died much more often than the women who were not examined. After watching this heartbreaking situation for three years, he established a new rule for his ward. He ordered every physician and medical student who had participated in autopsies of the dead to carefully wash his hands before examining living maternity patients.

In April 1847, before the new rule went into effect, fifty-seven (or one out of six) women had died in Dr. Semmelweis's ward. Then he instituted the hand-washing rule. In June, only one out of every forty-two women died. In July, only one out of every eighty-four women died. This is a fourteen-fold decrease in mortality! These astonishing statistics strongly indicated that fatal infections had been carried from corpses to living patients.

One day, after performing autopsies and washing their hands, the physicians and students entered the medical ward and examined a row of beds containing twelve women. Eleven of the twelve women quickly developed temperatures and died.

Another new thought was born in Semmelweis's alert brain: some mysterious element was evidently carried from one living patient to others, and with fatal consequences. Logically, Selmmelweis ordered that everybody wash his hands carefully after examining each living patient. Immediately, howls of protest were raised against the "nuisance"

> of washing, washing, washing; but the mortality rate went further down.
>
> Was Semmelweis acclaimed by his fellows? To the contrary, lazy students, prejudiced obstetricians, and jealous superiors scorned and belittled him so much that he was dismissed from the hospital. His successor threw out the washbasins and up shot the mortality rate to the old terrifying figures. Were his colleagues convinced then? Not at all. Even the world-renowned pathologist Rudolf Verchow continued to ridicule Semmelweis. We mortals might as well face it; our heads are so hardened by pride and prejudice that proof can rarely penetrate them (50).

The necessity of hand washing is a principal that God gave to Moses thirty-five hundred years ago to prevent the spread of disease.

Doctors throughout history have shunned this principal in part, even when introduced by brilliant experimenting minds. They now accept the part about washing their hands.

Albumin is involved in just about everything your body does. According to scientist Kenneth Seeton, a person's albumin count is the prime factor in determining health, (51) and Dr. Richard Gilleman has documented that a low Albumin count is connected to heart disease (51). The balance of Albumin should be at least 4.8 grams per liter. The average in the U.S. is 4.1. The average in Japan is 4.6.

That albumin count is connected to cleanliness – which is next to godliness - is a proven fact, according to Kenneth Seeton (51). However, every single medical doctor I have mentioned this to has come back with an arrogant response, in particular the Hepatologist. Upon suggesting to him the connection between an individual's Albumin count and wellness, his response in part was something like "that is the most ridiculous thing I've heard."

The thinking mind aligns the events of history with the words spoken by God and with seemingly new discoveries and then connects them.

I here and now inform you that the majority of people who are mentally equipped to become doctors, for the most part are so head strong and resistant to reality that they reside only in a cubical of education they received or are required to take.

The problem lies in the field. It's like a farmer. If he owns a field, he farms it. He doesn't cross over and farm something that isn't his. Doctors are indoctrinated in their learned behavior and allow in little else. History proves it, and the FDA is a prime example of this lunacy.

Harmless herbs are considered an expensive sewer additive by the most renowned doctors in the field of Hepatitis C. I'm sure not so many years will pass until these relics of the past will be regarded as fools of a dark age.

Kenneth Seeton also introduces the challenge that there are two minds. The mind of the immune system and the mind of the brain. When the immune system is overloaded it robs the ability of the mind to develop or function at full capacity, thus robbing you of your full IQ potential. If your antibody measure is being lowered to support your immune system defense, you have less for intellectual development. In order to have a higher IQ you need a purified brain, which results if you remove the overload on the immune system. One way to lower the overload is to wash your hands and fingernails with an antibiotic, four to twenty times a day (51).

The need for cleanliness brings us to the conclusion that Moses was more correct than we ever thought possible and it's all very scientific. For those of you who don't believe, consider, God is real.

Kenneth Seeton believes that eighty percent of diseases are transmitted through rubbing of the eyes and nose. Self-inoculated fingertips are the most effective way to transmit ear, nose and throat problems.

The albumin count cannot be raised by diet. The only way to bring the antibodies down is by removing infection from eyes and nose. To look at this in a more convincing way consider that one gram of albumin equals twelve trillion molecules.

If you wish to overcome Hepatitis C it is critical to follow the previous scenario absolutely in order to free up the immune system and to boost it to conquer your potentially fatal disease.

Remember, "You can't create Shakespeare in a dirty house."

The relation of albumin to health and cleanliness "is the largest discovery in Medical History" (51).

I suggest that we look at medicine as in transition, rather than factual, which is what the greatest alternative doctors gave to me.

We need to transition back to God as our good shepherd, who created everything and told us how to deal with all things. We have simply failed at studying, understanding and practicing his word. (Refer to Addendum 1 for additional information on Albumin)

Chapter Twenty-Five

Foods to Help You be Hepatitis C Free

Artichokes (Cynara Scolymus L.)

Artichokes are a native of the Mediterranean and a perennial in the thistle group, the same group as milk thistle. Dr. Finnegan prescribed two artichokes per day, preferably organically grown. I suggest you wash them thoroughly. The organic ones often have bugs, while the non-organic ones have insecticides. Many people feel that artichokes are too labor intensive. Be assured they are well worth the effort.

Artichokes also can be obtained marinated or plain in jars and cans. A typical can of artichoke hearts ranges in cost from $1.99 to $4.00. They make a great appetizer and are good in salads. If you like deep fried, batter them up, dump them in some good grease, and they are the best. There is also a company, De Boles, who produces pastas of all types made from the Jerusalem artichoke flower. They have macaroni and cheese, spaghetti, linguine, lasagna and all shapes and sizes of pasta. You can and should literally inundate your diet with every sort of artichoke replacement as much as possible. These products love your liver. They possess properties that clean and help restore liver function.

Jean Carper found:

> A series of studies in 1940 by a Japanese researcher found that the artichoke lowered total cholesterol somewhat, stimulated production of bile by the liver, performed as a diuretic, and enhanced 'well-being strikingly'.
>
> In 1969 French scientists were so successful in using artichoke extract for treating liver and kidney ailments that they took out a patent on it. In fact, cynarin, a constituent of the artichoke, was formulated into a drug lowering blood cholesterol. Cynarin also is well known to be "liver protective" (52).

Distilled Water

It is important that the Hepatitis C patient consume more than an average amount of water frequently throughout the day and night. I suggest that you keep a bottle of distilled water next to your bed and drink some each time you wake up through the night. This helps cleanse the liver by removing toxins and other unwanted substances. Drink your favorite water during the day.

Raw Eggs

Eat one raw egg per day. They are easy to digest and contain many enzymes and live food source nutrients that cooked eggs simply don't have. They are great in milk shakes or pop one in your slim fast.

Jean Carper continues:

Chickens have lots of rotavirus infections and the antigen - the viral agent that provides the pattern for the antibody - is similar to that of humans.

Dr. Yolken sees chickens as a virtual antibody factory. He notes that a single chicken could provide up to thirty kilograms of immunoglobin a year…Eggs have the potential of providing a large, economical supply of antibodies, fit for consumption by all ages (52).

Buckwheat

Buckwheat has been widely recognized as a great cleanser for the liver. You can incorporate it into pancakes instead of flour or wherever flour is needed. Also, in many health food stores, you can find cereals made from buckwheat.

Spinach

Spinach is prescribed as a preventive against hepatocellular carcinoma. Even though spinach is rich in iron, and we want to avoid iron, much of the iron in spinach is not absorbed because it is inside a cell membrane. This cell membrane often doesn't break down, and therefore passes through your system.

Several studies have indicated there are properties in spinach that help to prevent liver cancer.

Jean Carper found:

A new United States Department of Agriculture analysis finds that raw spinach has thirty-six milligrams of total arotenoids per hundred grams; where as raw carrots have fourteen milligrams per hundred grams, most of it in beta-carotene. Although beta-carotene is a confirmed cancer antagonist, spinach's panoply of other carotenoids may possess anti-cancer activity, and may be even more responsible than beta-carotene for spinach's splendid showing in population surveys of cancer-preventive foods (52).

Foods that are recognized to be good for liver function.

Foods that are especially good for rebuilding the liver are: flax seeds, flax seed oil, beet tops, beets, artichokes, lemon juice, carrots, greens, whole grains, raw yogurt from good quality milk, organic liver and egg yolks.

The Hepatitis C patient needs to recognize that it is easy to overload on protein and soon your ammonia level starts going up. That can get you in big trouble in terms of your central nervous system.

The few doctors who recommend a diet for there Hepatitis C patients suggest the elimination of all fried foods, red meat, alcohol, and coffee, while emphasizing cooked vegetables and grains along with limited amounts of chicken, fish, and turkey.

Yogurt; The Super-Immune Booster.

I consumed yogurt daily during my recovery period, and still do. There are many wonderful properties about yogurt that I had no knowledge of. The following are some of them.

Dr. Khem Shahani found:

"Lactobacillus acidophilus DDS-, enhance immune function by eliminating or inhibiting the formation of cancer-causing chemicals. Nitrates, commonly used in food processing, can be converted via enzymes to carcinogenic nitrosamines in the gut. Lactobacillus acidophilus is able to halt this process first by reducing the quantity of potential carcinogens, and second by deactivating certain cancer-causing enzymes, especially d-glucrondase and b-glucosidase.

The "Benefits of Yogurt," a report published in the *Journal of Immunotherapy,* found that acidophilus containing yogurt eaten over several months increased gamma-interferon, an important immune-enhancing protein that prevents viruses from reproducing themselves. Also noted was a reduction in inflammatory responses of the gut. IgE, an immunoglobulin that is effective in destroying parasites, is enhanced when lactobacillus bulgaricus was added to the diet. It was found to have powerful antibacterial properties, allowing IgE to function optimally(53).

Chapter Twenty-Six

Things to Avoid

Homogenized, Pasteurized Dairy Products

Pasteurization of milk is simply the heating of milk to a high temperature for a period of time to kill certain bacteria. This heating process also destroys most of the essential elements of milk, basically making it relatively worthless to consume. You may have noticed that cooked milk often states on the side of the container that the producer has added vitamin D3 and vitamin A. Milk is produced by mothers for the nourishment of their young. This milk contains many essential nutrients, enzymes and other factors that are destroyed by heat.

"Homogenized milk is considered the number one cause of heart disease in the United States by Dr. Kurt Oster and many others" (54).

For those of you who weren't raised on a farm, I shall attempt to explain why Americans homogenize milk.

In raw milk the butterfat rises to the top of the milk. This amount of butterfat is just too much for the average American to deal with, so along came the process of homogenization. Put simply, homogenization combines the milk and the butterfat. Butterfat is surrounded by a special enzyme that aids in its' digestion. This enzyme is known by the initials "XO" which stands for Xanthine Oxidase.

Due to the results of homogenization, digestion of raw milk in the stomach only barely begins. Most of the fat digestion doesn't really start until in the upper intestine, and it finishes in the liver. The liver is made to handle the digestion and use of fat in our body.

If you drink raw milk, the butterfat with the XO enzyme goes into the stomach, then into the small intestine and finally into the liver. The liver breaks up the fat into what are called fatty acids, and the body uses them. When milk is homogenized, the butterfat is so small that is gets into the stomach and goes into the upper intestine. It is so small that it can pass right through the upper intestine and then into your body. "However, as this little particle of fat gets into your bloodstream, it will eventually go through the liver and get digested... Due to the liver being a filter, all the blood goes through the liver and gets cleaned" (54).

This process of homogenization causes an impaired liver to have to work harder to deal with this processed food. It is a completely unnatural food that the human body has never had to deal with until the twentieth century. Beyond stressing the impaired liver, "the homogenized fat gets into the bloodstream, it carries along with it the XO enzyme. Once the XO enzyme gets inside of an artery, it eats and attacks the inside of the artery wall" (54).

This doesn't just happen in milk. It happens with everything made from milk; cottage cheese, cheese, butter, sour cream, etc. Luckily we can now purchase raw milk and raw milk products in many states.

When I was a small boy I used to help my father milk the cows. He would pour the pails of milk in a red contraption called a separator. I would turn its large red handle and out one spout would come cream, and out the other, fat-free raw milk. We would then churn the cream into butter in a large round wooden cylinder with a stick coming out the top. We even made real ice cream with fresh, raw cream from cows that never thought of eating chicken manure or ever had a hormone shot. It sure tasted better than anything I can remember.

Hard Liquor

Liquor is hard on your liver. The best reason I can think of not to drink liquor is because if you are a drinker, the probability of receiving a liver transplant, if you ever need one, is slim to none. Also, consumption of large amounts of alcohol inflames the liver and for people with Hepatitis C, it usually makes you feel sicker, taking the fun out of it. It is best to at least minimize alcohol intake or better yet do away with it all together.

Sugar Substitutes (Saccharine, Equal, etc...)

It is my understanding that sugar substitutes, especially saccharine, require sixty times more effort by the liver to process them than to process sugar. Also, I suggest that the next time you go out to eat and see one of those little pink packages on the table, pick it up and read the back. It says in plain English, "This product has been shown to cause cancer…"Use honey and raw sugar instead.

Analysis shows nearly 100% of independent research finds problems with aspartame (NutraSweet).

> "An analysis of peer reviewed medical literature using MEDLINE and other databases was conducted by Ralph G. Walton, MD, Chairman, The Center for Behavioral Medicine, Professor of Clinical Psychiatry, Northeastern Ohio Universities College of Medicine. Dr. Walton analyzed 162 studies, which were felt to have relevance to Human safety question. Of those studies, 74 studies had aspartame Industry-sponsorship and 90 were funded without any industry money.
>
> Of the 90 non-industry-sponsored studies, 83 (92%) identified one or more problems with aspartame. Of the 7 studies that did not find a problem, 6 of those studies were conducted by the FDA. Given that a number of FDA officials went to work for the aspartame Industry immediately following approval (including the former FDA Commissioner), many consider these studies to be equivalent to industry-sponsored research.
>
> Of the 74 aspartame industry-sponsored studies, all 74 (100%) claimed that no problems were found with aspartame. This is reminiscent of tobacco industry research where it is primarily the tobacco research that never finds problems with

the product, but nearly all of the independent studies do find problems.

The 74 aspartame industry industry-sponsored studies are those, which one invariably sees cited in PR/news reports and reported by organizations funded by Monsanto/Benevia/NutraSweet (e.g., IFIC, ADA).

These studies have serve design deficiencies which help guarantee the "desired" outcomes" (55).

Medical Doctors

The people who attach M.D. to their name should be avoided completely during your healing process. Hopefully after reading my book, you can understand why I feel the way I do. If, for some reason you cannot, here are a few more reasons. They are very expensive, and they know nothing about curing Hepatitis C. They do know how to prescribe Interferon but you don't want to take Interferon until the last resort. Finally, if you get to the point of a liver transplant, then of course medical doctors are the only resource. I only hope you pick one who is a good mechanic, and one who has a good supply of livers.

Reason number two; Nov. 29 1999---In a blistering report released Monday, a prestigious medical group said America's entire health care system needs "dramatic changes" to cut the enormous number of deaths and injuries from medical errors.

THE GROUP SAID hospitals should report mistakes to the federal government, not keep them secret as they often do now.

"For too long medical errors in hospitals and elsewhere have been buried and it is long overdue that they need to be reported to public agencies," said Dr. Sid Wolfe of Public Citizen, a consumer watchdog group.

Experts say between 44,000 and 98,000 Americans die from mistakes every year in hospitals alone. That makes hospital errors the eighth leading cause of death---actually ahead of traffic accidents, breast cancer and AIDS.

The report from the Institute of Medicine, a division of the National Academy of Sciences, said the numbers could be cut sharply. It sets as "a minimum goal a 50 percent reduction in errors over five years."

"The medical profession seems to like to keep the errors that are made a secret to maintain the faith in the profession," said attorney Andrew Meyer" (56).

This article was reported in USA Today, the Washington Post and the New York Times, all on the front page. The L A Times refers to the story on page 3.

How many occupations do you know of that can kill 98,000 people a year and not have it hit the headlines for decades? 98,000 are just short of **DOUBLE the number of Americans killed in Vietnam.** (For additional information on medical doctors refer to Addendum 2).

Hydrogenated Oil

Dr. John Finnegan warns:

> More than 200 million people may have been killed by refined oils. More people may have been killed from the harmful effects of refined oils and the deficiency of Omega-3 fatty acids than have been killed by all the wars of the century.
>
> Many people are greatly concerned about the continuing increase in degenerative disease today. They understand that there is a connection between our consumption of refined and hydrogenated oils – including those contained in margarine and many processed foods - and the breakdown of our health and immune systems (57).

It is nearly impossible to buy a cookie, cracker, cake, bread, donut or pastry, and the list goes on, that does not contain hydrogenated oil. Dr. Ed Wagner told me that it could take six to nine months for hydrogenated oil to pass through the liver, thus acting as a literal poison.

Stress

It is hard to say, "avoid stress", especially when your doctor has just announced that you have Hepatitis C and you are going to die a horrible death. You give up the idea of ever receiving a liver transplant when he tells you that forty people die waiting for a liver transplant for every one who gets one. Then he says imagine yourself well, but also make sure your will is in order. He then sends you on your way with a prescription for Interferon, which will no doubt cause you to beat your mate, hate your children and kill your dogs. Stress may seem minor compared to being subjected to this scenario, which I can tell you is not exaggerated.

Livers don't like stress. So buy a lotto ticket and dream at least a few minutes a day, just to escape reality for a little while. The body is not designed to deal with stress for more than short periods of time. Stress breaks down the immune system and that's what we want to boost. Read my book again and again, that should greatly relieve stress. Consult a spiritual advisor. Enjoy life!

Another great way to relieve stress is to construct a full, life-size replica of the doctor who gave you the blood transfusion that is now killing you. Hang it up and beat it. Or, if you are into guns, take it to a safe place to shoot and blow the living daylights out of it.

If that is just short of relieving your stress, drench it in gasoline and burn it. I suggest doing this in a fire safe environment and keep a fire extinguisher handy so you can put out the fire before it is completely disintegrated. Then you can urinate on the remains.

For those of you who are of a more conservative nature, please keep in mind, there are those of us who need extreme measures for success.

Prayer is good, and it works. Consult your pastor and have your church include you in the intercessory prayer meetings.

Take time out from your schedule and do something you don't usually do. If you like Bob Dylan, go to a Dylan concert.

EAT CHOCOLATE! Chocolate is a mild mood elevator and a good antioxidant.

Summary

In essence, remember that no two people react exactly the same way to any medicine, herb or group of herbs. You need to be intuitive and sense your inner being: develop a sensitivity of your being and experience the response. And keep uppermost in your mind that you can and must take responsibility for your health. You can adjust your life and health course better than anyone else can.

The quality of the herbs and supplements, how they are grown and processed determines how much benefit your body will receive from them.

It is not just the herb or supplement that is healing you. It is your immune system that monitors and protects your body. You must fuel your immune system with what it needs to do the job.

Liver cells degenerate in Hepatitis C and B in a similar fashion. The damage done to the liver is actually caused by the immune system reaction to the virus.

The immune system sends special immune cells, equipped with powerful chemicals to the liver. The virus is able to *hide* inside the liver cells. Because of this the virus is able to survive the immune cells attack.

Macrophages and Kupffer cells are sent to the liver by the immune system to release their chemicals to destroy the virus. The liver cells are exposed and become the unintended victim. Cirrhosis and cell death follows.

Peptides are the tiniest of protein molecules. They are found in live cell thymus and live cell liver as well as other live cell glandulars. Peptide growth factors actually communicate with the other cells in an organ. To simplify, they actually orchestrate the immune systems attack. They communicate with each other and alter their own behavior. These peptides actually convey information inside their animal host.

Mucopolysaccharides are found in properly prepared aloe vera, reishi mushrooms, and shark cartilage.

Dr. John Finnegan, N.D. states:

> "These 'leaders' (polysaccharides), the betaglucomannans have a unique penetrating action which acts as a biological vehicle drawing nutrients through the tissues and cells of the body. They actually penetrate the cell wall and become incorporated into the cell wall, carrying with them the body's own immune cell fighting mechanism" (44).

This process takes time and requires dedication. It is necessary to help support the liver function through proper diet, the elimination of toxic material, boosting the immune system through proper nutrition and protecting the liver during this process by consuming the herbs, foods and supplements discussed in this book.

The suggestions I make in this book work better than anything currently offered to you by the FDA for the treatment of Hepatitis C.

Testimonials

The following is feedback I have gotten from my readers. I hope that these testimonials will inspire hope in Hep. C sufferers and instill the determination necessary for your survival.

Client 1: This 40 year-old female started my program on November 3rd, 1999 after having been diagnosed with chronic Hepatitis C. Her blood tests at USC University Hospital showed that her ALT & AST levels were only slightly elevated but her viral load was over 1 million and she was anemic. She complained of significant hair loss, irritability, rashes and a general feeling of discontent, naseousness and depression. After starting my program she still complained about numerous problems, however, I attribute these problems to her use of Interferon. On March 1st, 2000 she faxed PCR quantification HCV RNA by PCR QUANT showing <3.3 HCV non-detected. "Thanks to you and your nutritional supplements, along with Interferon & Rebitol therapies, I no longer have HCV." She no longer experiences the rashes, sickness, nauseous ness, and her hair has grown back.

Client 2: This 37 year-old male had completed 1 year of Interferon/Ribavirin, which failed. He started my program on March 15, 2000. His tests read HCV ULTRAQUANT-SPECIALTY HEP C VIRUS RNA ULTRA showing a viral load of 953,710. His ALT was 61 while the normal range is 0-38. His AST was 40 with a normal count range at 0-40. He followed my program precisely and a blood test 30 days later on April 14, 2000 showed his viral load at 246,600. This is a 75% drop! His ALT went down to 18 and his AST down to 33. He called often and followed my program precisely for 30 days. He then went to china town and was told some of the components of my program could be reproduced for less money. His 60 day test reveled that his liver enzymes and viral load rose again.

Client 3: 49 year-old male tried Interferon / Ribavirin combo therapy for 6 months prior to starting my program. His viral load was more than 1 million and was actually higher when he ended the combo therapy than when he started. His AST was 88 (1-37 normal), ALT was 165 (1-42 normal). He started my program February on 20, 2000 and his next blood test dated April 21, 2000 showed a significant drop in his viral load to 742, 047. His AST went down to 30 and his ALT dropped to 44. This client reported feeling much better, having more energy, and was back to feeling ambitious again.

Client 4: This 56 year-old male tried 1 year of the combo therapy and it failed. His Viral Load was at 220,000, ALT 166 (1-50), and AST 97 (0-45). He indicated that he had been extremely sick, fatigued, and nauseous during Interferon treatment. He also stated that Interferon caused him feelings of hostility, aggressive behavior and caused him to perform acts that were outside of his character. I received a call from his wife only 30 days into my program in which she reported that his "baseball under the rib syndrome", which he had been experiencing for several years, was gone (swelling of the liver). At 6 weeks into my program he stated, "I feel better than I have in 10 years. I play golf 4 to 5 times per week!" A blood test 8 weeks later revealed similar numbers as his previous test but he stated, "I am not unhappy with the numbers. Even if they stayed the same I would much rather do this than Interferon." His test dated June 6, 2000 indicated that his numbers did eventually drop, his ALT down to 78, his AST to 61, and his Viral Load at 200,000. His doctor was happy with his improvement and told him that his liver was remodeling.

Client 5: 37 year-old Pharmacist started my program February 2000 after trying 6 months of the combo therapy. His wife called, informing that her husband was loosing weight and that his skin was pale gray in color. He was consistently fatigued, unable to work a full day, and his personality was fading. After just 2 weeks on my program another call from his wife confirmed that the color had returned to his skin and that he was feeling and acting somewhat healthier. A 30-day call reported that he had begun to gain weight and that his personality was back to the way he was when they were first married. He currently no longer feels sick, however, his blood tests indicated only a slight drop in his numbers (yet this information is reported form his doctor; Client 5 never saw his tests). This client continues on the program with great expectations. He stated that he would "rather see a Veterinarian for Hepatitis C than a doctor."

Client 6: wrote: "I was writing to you back in October and you were incredibly helpful and supportive. Besides wanting to thank you, I also want to give you an update. Since then my Viral Load has gone from 3,100,000 to 318,600-down 90% (depending how much one believes in that test). My AST went from 36 to 29 and ALT from 61 down to 43. All of this in less than 10 months! My feeling is that it is because of the Thymus, which is the only supplement besides Milk Thistle that I am diligent in taking every day. I could go on and on but I want to tell you how happy I was to look at the same doctor who told me there was NOTHING I could do besides Interferon to lower my counts and have him read my results now. Hope all is well with you and I was glad to see your web site up and running well."

Client7: wrote: "Lloyd, I just returned from yet another visit to the Lexington medical center, where a few weeks ago I had another Viral Count performed and guess what...I am clear of the virus! My doctor wants to do another count in 3 months to see if it is really true. I believe that the herbs really helped. He said if this was the same after 3 months that it was truly a miracle. Thought I would pass that on to you."

Client 8: Started on my program in August 1999. He had done a year of Interferon and the combo therapy and expressed anger and hostility beyond his imagination. He indicated that his desire to kill just about anything became an obsession. He reported his intolerance to his doctor and the doctor prescribed a tranquilizer, and a mood elevator. He was recently married and his wife, a registered nurse stayed with him; because she knew that it was the drug, not the man.

When he started my program he had been off the Interferon for 3 months. His viral load was 2,200,000. His ALT was 215 (normal range 0-40) and his AST was 210 (normal range 1-35). After 3 months he reported that his viral load dropped to less than one million, his ALT was 115 and his AST was 100. In February 2000 he reported that his viral load was less than 3.3 Hepatitis C non-detected. His ALT was 18 and his AST was 12. Client 8 reported to me that his doctor told him that he had the luck of experiencing a spontaneous remission.

Client 9: This 37 year-old male first called me in early Jan. 2000. He ordered my book and then showed it to his alternative doctor. He then ordered everything in my remedy.

He called several times for advice and was always reading and seeking every avenue for success. His ALT was at 160 (normal 11-66), his AST was 52 (normal 20-57) and his HCV RNA QUANT read 1.81 million.

As I learned about new products that showed success with Hepatitis C and added them to my website, this client would order them and use them as well.

He did a parasite cleanse and altered his diet in addition to making life style changes. This client even had his dental work redone to remove all of the metal from his mouth. He is truly a pleasure to work with.

He also saw a few different types of alternative doctors and did other therapies other than those discussed in Triumph Over Hepatitis C. In early August he faxed me his blood work showing normal counts! His AST was 24, his ALT was 43 and his HCV PCR QUANT went down to 350.000. That is down one million four hundred and fifty thousand in 8 months.

I cannot resist a little commentary. M.L. never doubted me nor did he ever question my integrity. He always made me feel like I was part of the family. He followed my program to the letter. (Blood Tests on file).

Just a few E-mails of over 20,000

"I just wanted to tell you how much I appreciate you making your story available on the Internet. When my husband was diagnosed with Hepatitis C, the first place I went was the net. I know that the AMA has only one objective; to keep their pockets filled while never "curing" anything. Although my uncle is head of Pathology at Penrose Hospital in Colorado Springs, and my husband's brother is a doctor in Chicago, I have learned that the best "drugs" for the human body are the natural ones. When my mom was diagnosed 5 years ago with PBC, I worked hard to get her to go to a naturopath, which she finally did and for the past 3 years her enzyme tests have been normal. She had a massive stroke in '75 and had been on so many drugs since then-no wonder her liver was compromised!

Have finished reading your book-what a nightmare you went through. I am glad that you are well now. When the GI doctor talked to us last week he, of course, said Interferon was the "only" treatment. I was armed with all the info from the net and asked him about natural herbal treatment, and this meek little man turned into a demon denouncing herbs and the fact that they are "not tested, regulated or pure" and that he wouldn't give "that stuff" to his own wife. I politely pointed out that all synthetic drugs pass through the liver and compromise it. He made a few more comments about the "efficacy" of Interferon, so I shut my mouth, realizing he was another closed-minded AMA robot. He wrote in my husband's records: "wife does not approve of treatment". GOOD! I want them to be aware that I am not going to stand by and watch these VA butchers kill my husband.

Sorry this is long winded. I am so grateful for all your research and compassion toward others that are suffering from this disease. I am confident that the information you have provided along with a good naturopath doctor, that my husband will be cured. Again, a great big Thanks!"

"I read, with great enthusiasm, your book on alternatives to the Interferon therapy. I am now recovering form the horrible effects of trying that therapy and want to start your program." C.H.

"I loved your book. You are a real wit!" S.S.

"I have not taken the medications the doctors want me to because I am so afraid of them. I chose to be on the herbs, Milk Thistle and Thymus that you suggested. Thank you for all your information and help. With people like you out there, life is still with us. Please keep me in your prayers as you are in mine. Lets beat this thing and help others beat it also." G.F.

"Hi, I started to read your book. There are so many interesting things and this is a book from one patient to other patients. This makes all the difference. I was shocked when I was reading that your health insurance canceled your policy. In Europe we don't have the same system and you can always go to the hospital, even when you are without a job. Keep up the good work." C.S.

"I absolutely loved your book! It is so inspiring, frank and hilarious. You have an excellent sense of humor that I completely understand." S.D.

"I have a lot of faith and I believe that it is not over for me. I have begun taking Aloe Vera, Liver Detox and Milk Thistle because I nearly died from the Interferon combination. I actually thought I was going to die before I got better and my doctor told me to keep on taking it. I couldn't even climb up the stairs because of weakness. My liver and my stomach swelled and I felt lousy. He told me that the herbs weren't proven when I told him my body wasn't agreeing with what he was saying. My stomach is still a little swollen but not as bad and I don't have any pain. I lead a natural active life and this diagnosis has been devastating, but your book has given me hope." A.W.

"Dear Lloyd,

I have been taking live thymus every other day for 6 weeks and following your book like it is the bible. Thank you so much for all of your help, time and effort." B.J.

"I have hepatitis C and have been through all the conventional treatments of Interferon. I initially had 6 months of injections of 3 million units 3 times per week. But my counts still weren't normal. My doctor referred me to the University of Florida Shands teaching hospital where Dr. Gary Davis was conducting a study for Shearing Plough. The study used the same treatment of 3 million units 3 times per week...when I still had high AST ALT levels, I was then given 5 million units 3 times week, until I developed such horrendous side effects that my doctor contacted Dr. Davis and had me removed from the study. When I stopped the study my AST was 128 and my ALT was 189. That was after several years of the Interferon combination treatment. During the course of this extended treatment I got mouth soars, lost most of my hair, was constantly exhausted and sick to my stomach, and I became increasingly depressed. I also saw things that were not there but in my case I had never experienced depression in my life and I am in my 50's. I now live with depression. I had been told that Interferon would leave your body once you stopped taking it. But in my case there seems to have been permanent damage to my brain pathways including the ones dealing with serotonin. It also affected my memory and I now have ADD. Since my liver is already in advanced cirrhosis I started taking Milk Thistle tablets as well as other parts of your program against my doctors advice. My ALT is now 32 and my AST 35. Of course my doctor still isn't convinced and won't be until it's proven by medical science that your program, instead of a spontaneous remission, healed me." S.H.

"Went home for lunch today and your book was on my kitchen table. Would have gotten back to you sooner but I couldn't put it down. I have already read it and it was SOO funny! It is great to see that you could preserve your sense of humor during such a crisis. Thanks again and it was great reading." A.L.

"I read your book and I really became enthusiastic over your method of healing. First, have my congratulations not only for your efforts to survive but also for strength of your faith and hope. To survive a serious accident followed by cancer and finally Hepatitis C is something extraordinary. Second, it made me happy to see that you had retained your sense of humor in those bad times; only a strong person is able to do that. I know I am not the first one telling you that your book, dealing with such a serious life-threatening problem like Hepatitis C in such a "smooth" and almost entertaining way is something particular. It gives enthusiasm to others suffering from the disease to try the same." T.S.

"Lloyd,

Wanted you to know that I have been on the program you suggested, plus a thymic formula from a Dr. Burgstiner in Georgia, for a few days short of 3 months. I got my first test results today and my ALT count has gone from 398 to 37 I want them to test for the virus but they haven't done that yet. Thanks for your help." J.H.

To J.H. from Lloyd

I would like to know if it would be all right with you if I print your E-mail of June 29 on my message board? I will remove your name and E-mail address and just leave your initials.

Please let me know.

Thank You

Lloyd

Lloyd,

I would have no problem with that. I feel so great after getting some positive results that I want everyone to know. I went through the same thing you did with the combination therapy of Interferon and Ribavirin. It got so bad that I couldn't even brush my own hair. I still have trouble with my mood swings but I am more positive than I have been in a long time and I hope that will help. Thanks for your help. J.H.

Dear Lloyd

If it wasn't for you I don't know where I would be. I could not think straight, I could not drive, and it was horrible. Now life is wonderful! One month on your program and I drove 8 hours to Maine and I didn't even get tired. Then I went to Colorado and went skiing for the first time in years. I can't thank you enough. After 60 days, my viral load has dropped from **663,260** to less than **100,780**. You are such an inspiration to me and I pray for you every night. G.H.

Dear Lloyd,

Excellent book! It works well for individuals looking for the kind of help you offer. I am recommending it to all of my Hepatitis patients.

Sincerely, J.M.T., M.D.

Lloyd,

After reading your book, I began taking Milk Thistle and drinking teas. In two months my ALT dropped from 103 to 44. My AST also dropped from 130 to 76 and I haven't touched any Interferon. Lloyd, your book has been the best inspiration for me. I'm sure I'll be talking to you again soon.

I am impressed, you're **THE MAN!** G.N.

"I've seen my dear friend go from standing on death's door to being a vital and healthy man again. He did it by following a program that he has since written into his book, Triumph Over Hepatitis C. Having been in the rock and roll business in the crazy 70's, I witnessed a lot of abusive behavior by people I admired. Some of those people are no longer with us but many of them, like Eric Clapton (who's band I was in for 4 years), turned their lives around and totally cleaned up their acts. Without the help that's available to people who need it and ask for it, I doubt many of us would have succeeded. For alcoholics and drug addicts there is AA and NA, and various other support groups. For people with Hepatitis C there is good proven advice in Lloyd Wright's book. If you know anyone who is suffering from this devastating health problem, before you even go near Interferon, try everything else you can to help-including getting this book for them. As I have seen in my friend, it WORKS! Sincerely**, Yvonne Elliman"**

Dear Lloyd,

I am writing to share my success and thank you for your work with the HCV.

I am 48 years old. Although I did some wild and crazy things in the 70's, for the past 20 years I have maintained a lifestyle of healthy living.

This summer I applied for a life insurance policy. Imagine my surprise and shock when I was denied coverage due to testing positive for the HCV.

I went to the Web and read stories of doom and gloom from the medical community. Then I visited your site! I ordered your book immediately.

In the meantime, I went to my family doctor who blew this off as "no big deal." He said it was like being on a slow moving train on a long track, that I would probably live with it, rather than die from it. He said I should probably have a follow up in about a year and gave me the name of a Gastroenterologist.

Your book came and I read it the first night. I ordered the supplements right away, tried to follow your regime as closely as possible, including the NatCell Thymus, which as you know is very expensive.

I went to the Gastroenterologist and he wanted me to start Interferon. I said, "No, it's not really known to work". He agreed. He wanted to schedule me for a liver biopsy. I said, "No, its not really going to alter my course". He said, "Start taking milk thistle, it's the only known thing to work. He didn't say how much to take or where to get it. That was O.K. I already knew.

I had been on the supplements for about a week when I went to my Chiropractor. He said to me, "I don't know what it is, but you're putting your body through some tremendous changes". That's when I told him about the HCV and starting the homeopathic supplements. He altered his technique that day to work on the area of the spine that controls the liver function.

I am happy to report that after only 5 weeks of your therapy in combination with my chiropractor, my SGOT (AST) has decreased from 86 to 38 (a reduction of 56% and in some lab reference ranges considered to be within the normal). My SGPT (ALT) has decreased from 112 to 54 (a reduction of almost 52%). Viral load was not drawn on the first set of labs so I have no baseline, but on the second lab draw my viral load was 8,000.

I recently added milk thistle and mushroom teas to my regime. I plan to have my labs drawn every three months, the next one around mid-November. I will let you know the results, but again expect to beat this. Again, thank you for sharing your work.

Sincerely, Al

References

1. "Placebos and Positive Belief Help Healing", *Hepatitis Alert*, Hepatitis Foundation International, Fall 1998, page 5.
2. Informational and Solicitation Letter from the American Liver Foundation, 1998.
3. Marohn, Stephanie "Naomi Judd, For the Country Queen, Alternative Medicine Rules" Alternative *Medicine Digest*, Issue 21, January 1998, pages 68-72.
4. U.S. News on CNN Internet, August 23, 1997, page 3.
5. Los Angeles Times, Part B Metro, February 23, 1994, page 3.
6. Satchell, Michael and Hedges, Stephen *U.S. News and World Report Online*, Sept 1, 1997, page 3.
7. Hall, Carl T. "Scientist Stalk a Quiet Killer, Sci Clone, Chiron Seek Hepatitis C Treatment," *San Francisco Chronicle*, July 21, 1995.
8. Genesis 2:29, King James Bible.
9. Phone conversation with Pat Conely 6/11/99. For further information contact: Price-Pottenger Nutrition Foundation, P.O. Box 2614 La Mesa, CA 91943-2614, 619-574-7763 or www.PRICE-Pottenger-org.

10. Rohrer, Jean "Healing Light: Milk Thistle", Internet, Pages 1-3.

11. Whitaker, Julian "Longevity Science Biopro Thymic Protein A", *Health and Healing*, March 1997.

12. Radchenko VG, Mitrofanova T, Serebriakova VI Vinogradova GL. The efficacy of immunomodulating preparations in treating patients with chronic cholestatic liver disease. Vrachebnoe Delo. 1992 Nov-Dec, (11-12): 38.

13. Berkow R, and Flectcher AJ. The Merck Manual of Diagnosis and Merck Research Laboratories, Rathway, NJ. 1992, 308.

14. Fausto, N.; Laird, A.D.; Webber, EH. "Liver regeneration. Role of growth factors and cytokines in hepatic regeneration." Journal of FASEB. 9(15): 1527-1536, Dec. 1999.

15. Teir, H. and Ravanti, K Experimental Cell Research. 5:500, 1953.

16. Blomqvist, K. Acta Path. Microbiol. Scaand, Suppl. 121, 1957.

17. Levi, J.U. and Zeppa, R.J. Surgical Research. 12: 114, 1972.

18. Compagno, J. and Grisham, J. Western Federal Proceedings32: 837,1973.

19. Lloyd, E.A.; Crozier, N.; Pamphlet, G.; Wells, M.; Saunders, S.J. British Journal of Experimental Pathology. 55:251, 1974.

20. Starzl, T.E.; Terblanche, J.; Porter, K.A.; Jones, A.F.; Usui, S.; Mazzoni, G. "Growth-stimulating factor in regenerating canine liver." The Lancet. January 20, 1979, pp. 127-130.

21. Michalopoulos, G.K. Journal of FASEB. 4:176-187, 1990.

22. Russell, W.E. and DuBois, R.N. in Liver Disease in Children. (Suchy, F.J. and Craven, L., Eds.) (St. Louis: Mosby, 1994), pp. 11-30.

23. LaBrecque, D. American Journal of Gastroenterology. 69:S86S96, 1994.

24. Sporn, M.B. and Roberts, A.B. Peptide growth factors and inflammation, tissue repair and cancer." Journal of Clinical Investigation. 78:329-332, 1986.

25. Sporn, M.B. and Roberts, A.B. "Peptide growth factors are multifunctional." Nature. 332:217-219.

26. Barkai, A. and McQuaid, C. "Predator-prey role reversal in a marine benthic ecosystem." Science. 242:62-64, 1988.

27. Sehgal, P.B.; May, L.T.; Tamm, I.; Vilcek, J. "Human Beta-2 interferon and B-cell differentiation factor BSF-2 are identical." Science. 235:731-732, 1987.

28. Kishimoto, T. and Hirano, T. "Molecular regulation of 6lymphocyte response," Annual Review of Immunology. 6:485-512, 1988.

29. Nimer, S.D.; Champlin, R.E.; Golde, D.W. "Serum cholesterol lowering activity of

granulocyte-macrophage colony-stimulating factor." Journal of the American Medical Association. 260:3297-3300, 1988.

30. Saito, H.; Ebinuma, H.; Tada, S.; Tsunematsu, S.; Atsukawa, K.; Masuda, T.; Tsuchiya, M.; Ishii, H. "Enhancing effect of the liver extract and flavin adenine Dinucleotide mixture on anti-viral efficacy of interferon in patients with chronic hepatitis C." Keio Journal of Medicine. 45(l): 48-53, March 1996.

31. Ibid

32. Nelson, C.; Moffat, B.; Jacobsen, N.; Henzel, W.J.; Stults, J.T.; King, K.L.; McMurtrey, A.; Vandlen, R.; Spencer, S. "Giycerophosphoryiethanolamine (GPEA) identified as an hepatocyte growth stimulator in liver extracts." Experimental Cell Research. 229(l): 20-26, Nov. 1996.

33. Akatsu, T.; Nagata, N.; Kugai, N.; Yasutomo, Y.; Kinoshita, T.; Kosano, H.; Takaatani, 0.; Takishima, K.; Mamiya, G. "On the activities of parathyroid hormone-like factor and transforming growth factors in extract of pancreatic cancer associated with humoral hypercalcemia of malignancy." Acta Endocrinology (Copenhagen). 118(2): 232-238, June 1988.

34. Ueno, N.; Baird, A.; Esch, F.; Shimasaki, S.; Ling, N.; Guillemin, R. "Purification and partial characterization of mitogenic factor from bovine liver: structural homology with basic fibroblast

growth factor." Regulation Pept, 16(2): 135-145, Dec. 1986.

35. Rodriguez-Fragoso, L. "Physiologic and physiopathologic role of hepatocyte growth factor." Review of Investigational clinics, 50(4): 355-367, July/Aug. 1998.

36. Balkovetz, D.F. and Lipschutz, J.H. "Hepatocyte growth factor and the kidney: it is not just for the liver." International Review of Cytology. 186:225-260, 1999.

37. Matsumoto, K. and Nakamura, T. "HGF: its organotrophic role and therapeutic potential." Ciba Foundation Symposium. 212:198-211, 1997.

38. Michalopoulos, G.K. and DeFrances, M.C. "Liver regeneration." Science. 276(5309): 60-66, Apr. 4 1997.

39. Law, David "Medical Mushrooms: An Ancient Alternative to Synthetic Drugs, A Positive Approach to Health and Wellness", Internet, pages 1-3.

40. Packer, Ester "Alpha-Lipoic Acid: The Universal Antioxidants", 1997, pages 2-3.

41. Mowrey, Dan "Licorice for the Female Reproduction System "Health Store News, June/July 1995.

42. Lust, John The Herb Book Bantam Books, New York, 1974, page 171.

43. Davis, Brent W. "A New World Class Herb for A. K. Practice", Summer 1992.

44. Finnegan N.D. Dr. John Excerpts from "The Healing Aloe: Nature's Wondrous Gift and Cancer Prevention and Recovery: A Nutritional Approach."

45. John C. Pittman, M.D. Immune Enhancing Effects Of Aloe.

46. Larsen, Hans R. "Vitamin C: Your Ultimate Health Insurance" International Health News.

47. Carper, Jean "Vitamin C" Chapter in The Food Pharmacy, Bantam Books, N.Y., 1999, page 222.

48. Schiff Supplement Facts, page 1.

49. Exodus 15:26, King James Bible.

50. McMillan, S.I. None of these Diseases, Fleming H Rand Company, Old Tappan, NI. 1984, pages 24-25.

51. The Tony Brown Journal, The T.V. Series, Show # 1615, "The Life Factor", 1996.

52. Carper, Jean The Food Pharmacy, Bantam Books, N.Y., 1988, pages 105,121and 279.

53. Shahani and Fernandes. 1990. "Anticarcinogenic and immunological properties of dietary lactobacilli," Journal of Food Protection 53: 704-1.

54. Oster, Kurt "Milk: The Homogenization Deception", Internet, 1999.

55. Aspartame / NutraSweet News Release. October 17, 1996 Aspartame (NutraSweet) Toxicity Information Center.

56. Bazell, Robert " Medical errors a major killer." N B C NEWS NOV.29, 1999.

57. Finnegan, N.D., Dr. John "The Shocking Truth about Refined Oils", Health Naturally, August/September 1994, page 20.

58. Heyman, Dr. Jeri L., Ph.D., "The Secret Promise Of Aloe Vera", Herbal Answers Inc.

59. Walker, Dr. Morton.

Appendix A

Informational Article about Interferon alpha –2b recombinant

American Liver Foundation

INFORMATION

The Liver in Health and Disease

HEPATITIS C: THERAPY

Gary L. Davis, MD
University of Florida
Gainesville, Florida

Key Points:

1. Chronic hepatitis C is a heterogeneous disease whose natural history and response to treatment is probably influenced by multiple factors including but not limited to viral genotype, level of viral replication, and histology.

2. Interferon is the only agent of proven efficacy in the treatment of Hepatitis C. Standard treatment is Interferon alfa-2b at a dose of three million units three times a week. The initial course of treatment is 6 months, but nearly all patients relapse and require re-treatment. The goal of Interferon treatment is suppression of active disease; this usually requires long-term therapy. Eradication of virus does not appear to be a realistic goal in most patients.

3. Higher doses and longer duration of initial therapy have limited benefit over standard therapy. However, higher initial doses may increase the interval before relapse and escalation of the dose may achieve response in some non-responders.

4. Treatment trials have tended to study relatively homogenous patient groups and the possibility of extrapolating these results to different patient populations is extremely limited. This is especially true of studies from geographic areas. Thus, future studies should: (1) consider genotype, viral load, and histology in stratification; and (2) include a control group of standard treatment for comparison.

5. Selection of patients for this chronic treatment remains controversial. Treatment of patients with active disease is most cost- effective, but other factors such as the degree of symptoms must be considered.

6. The definition of response to treatment is evolving as a technology of measurement of HCV improves. It is likely that future treatment strategies will be dependent

upon virologic endpoints in addition to, or instead of, serum ALT.

7. Different agents and adjuncts have been incompletely studied to date. Ribavirin reduces serum ALT levels to normal and improves fatigue in nearly half of patients. Histology and virus levels do not appear to be significantly altered. The mechanism of its action of this interesting agent is not clear.

INTRODUCTION

The first trial of interferon as therapy for chronic non-A, non-B hepatitis was reported in 1986. This pilot study demonstrated that alpha Interferon therapy: (1) was effective at low doses (in comparison to doses previously shown to be required for hepatitis B and D); (2) decreased serum ALT levels promptly upon initiation of therapy, a pattern suggestive of an antiviral effect of Interferon; and (3) was usually associated with relapse when treatment was stopped, indicating a failure to eradicate the virus. Many subsequent controlled studies have now confirmed all of these original observations. A dose of 3 million units of recombinant Interferon alfa-2b thrice weekly for 6 months is the currently approved standard for initial therapy in the United States. With the discovery of the hepatitis C virus responsible for non-A, non-B hepatitis and the availability of moderately sensitive techniques for detaching the virus, it is now apparent that the biochemical response to Interferon (normalization of ALT) is associated with loss of detectable viremia; thus, the primary response of Interferon is indeed due to the antiviral effects of the drug. However, the high relapse rate confirms the earlier suspicion that interferon is usually unable to eradicate the virus, which persists at levels below the current limits of detection in serum, liver, or peripheral blood mononuclear cells.

It is apparent that the usual effect of Interferon in patients with chronic Hepatitis C who respond to this therapy is one of viral suppression, not eradication or cure. Sustained or prolonged response to treatment (persistently normal ALT levels) occurs in only 15-20% of patients and is often associated with detectable viremia despite the biochemical absence of apparent hepatic injury. The observations from these early studies are important and must be considered in establishing appropriate justification and goals for Interferon therapy in clinical practice. Several crucial points must be made:

1. Interferon therapy appears to eradicate or cure infection in only a small proportion of patients. Thus, cure is an unrealistic goal of current Interferon regimens.

2. Interferon is suppressive to the Hepatitis C virus. The goal of therapy should be to suppress infection to a degree that liver disease is minimized.

3. The currently approved regimen of therapy (3 million units 3x per week for 6 months) is sub-optimal. It should be considered as initial therapy, not as definitive therapy. The goal of chronic viral suppression will require prolonged therapy, re-treatment of relapse, or maintenance regimens

Currently, clinical and basic research in Hepatitis C is just beginning to shed light on the issues important to therapeutics in this confusing disease. It is now apparent that the disease course is only slowly progressive in most patients; thus, histology may be important in assessing the timing of therapeutic investigation. It is evident that the natural history is different between genotypes. The initial and long-term response to therapy is also affected by both genotype and the level of viremia.

The differences in response to Interferon therapy, which occur as a result of viral differences, are critical to clinical research in therapeutics. Literally dozens of studies of various interferon dose regimens have appeared to demonstrate superiority of every conceivable permutation of dosing to the currently accepted regimens. However, few have compared these novel and potentially useful regimens to standard dosing. Since genotypes are geographically diverse and have significant influence on response to interferon, trials conducted on one continent or even in different countries of regions within a continent are not comparable. Changes in therapeutic regimens from the current standard must be based on careful comparisons of different regimens among genotypically similar patients with similar viral loads. It is likely that a single dosing strategy is not appropriate for all patients. Differences in the Hepatitis C virus from country to country may warrant local modifications in interferon dosing. Unfortunately, this implies that the considerable effort and expense of clinical trials may have little applicability outside of the area where they are conducted. At a bare minimum, genotype and the degree of viremia need to be considered as stratification levels in designing future clinical trials.

Finally, the traditional marker for assessing treatment response is normalization of the serum ALT level. Although this endpoint was established before identification of the Hepatitis C virus, it appears to be as appropriate as measuring HCV-RNA for determining the initial response to Interferon, i.e. normalization of ALT is usually associated with loss of detectable virus from the serum. However, after discontinuation of Interferon, HCV-RNA usually becomes detectable well before re-evaluation of ALT (the traditional definition of relapse) occurs. In fact, viremia may be present for months to years after Interferon is stopped despite persistently normal ALT levels ("sustained remission"). Other markers include aGST, procollagen III, and chocolate clearance, are under study and may serve as adjunctive markers of response. Clearly, future studies should consider alternative markers of response and relapse, which might prove to be more clinically useful than those currently employed.

TREATMENT OF CHRONIC HEPATITIS C

Standard Therapy

Standard initial therapy for chronic Hepatitis C infection is recombinant Interferon alfa-2b at a dose of 3 x 106 units administered subcutaneously 3 times per week for 6 months. This regimen is based on the results of 3 randomized controlled trials, which employed an identical protocol and were conducted in France and the United States. These trials demonstrated that 41% of patients normalized the serum ALT level during treatment and 70% of responders had histological improvement. Response to treatment is greatest in those patients without advanced inflammation or cirrhosis, high HCV-RNA levels, of genotypes 1a and 1b (Simmonds). Almost all responders (normal ALT) lose detectable HCV-RNA by reverse transcription polymerase chain reaction (RT-PCR) by the end of therapy. However, relapse occurs in 50-70% of patients after the end of the initial course and is associated with return of detectable HCV-RNA. Relapse usually responds to re-treatment with Interferon.

Alternative regimens: Higher dose, Longer duration.

The best way to improve the efficacy of interferon treatment is to improve the initial response and its durability. Controlled trials of alternative regimens including higher doses, daily dosing or longer durations of therapy have not shown that these schedules improve the response rate. However, higher doses of Interferon may increase the durability of the initial response, i.e. reduce early relapse. The effect of tapering the dose after the initial 6 months on subsequent relapse is unclear, having been reported to either reduce or have no effect on relapse. These findings need to be confirmed.

Adjuncts to Interferon Therapy & Combination Therapy

Several compounds have been suggested to improve the response to Interferon in patients with chronic hepatitis C. Ursodeoxycholic acid has been proposed as either a single agent or adjunct to Interferon, but its effects on viral replication and inflammation have been incompletely examined. NSAIDS have a potential role in augmenting the antiviral effects of Interferon through their ability to block prostaglandin synthesis, increase the epoxygenase pathway, and increase 2', 5' oligoadenylate synthetase, one of the effectors of Interferon activity. These effects have not been proven in vivo. N-acetyl cysteine (NAC), an antioxidant and glutathione source, has been shown in one pilot study to induce response to interferon when patients had previously failed to respond. However, most patients with chronic Hepatitis C are not glutathione deficient and the therapy is expensive and distasteful. Controlled trials need to determine if NAC has any effects in chronic Hepatitis C.

Ribavirin has not proven to significantly increase response to interferon in a single published study. However, several pilots studies published in abstract form suggest a possible effect. This agent's role has only begun to be explored. No scientific rationale exists for prednisone pretreatment in chronic Hepatitis C. Corticosteroids increase HCV replication. Nonetheless, prednisone pre-treatment has been shown in one study in the Orient to increase the durability of response. These findings need to be reexamined in a controlled fashion in genotyped patients.

Alternatives to Interferon

There are few alternatives to interferon on the horizon for patients with HCV infection. Thymosin is not effective. Ribavirin shows some promise as a single agent in the treatment of chronic Hepatitis C, but its effects are difficult to interpret. Although ribavirin is a nucleoside analogue and know antiviral agent, its ability to normalize serum ALT levels and improve symptoms in patients with chronic HCV infection does not appear to result from inhibition of HCV (viral levels remain unchanged). It is possible that the agent acts through inhibition of some effectors of tissue damage. Certainly, clarification of the mechanism of action of this agent will help define the pathogenesis of hepatic injury in HCV infection.

PROBLEMS WITH TREATMENT OF CHRONIC HEPATITIS C:

Interferon therapy of chronic HCV infection is not straight-forward. Therapy is initially effective in only a portion of patients and it appears that eradication of infection is unusual in patient infected with the genotypes most common in the United States and most areas of Europe. Thus, several issues are important in understanding the appropriateness and limitations of Interferon treatment.

Selection of Patients

Treatment of patients should be directed at those who will benefit from the intervention. Several issues are important to defining this benefit: cost, durability for response, and natural history of disease. In the case of HCV infection, interferon treatment is effective in only about 40%. Since response is usually not permanent, re-treatment and perhaps long-term maintenance therapy is required to maintain control of the disease. Natural history studies have shown that HCV is a slowly progressive disease and that patients at greatest risk of progression are those with moderate to severe periportal inflammation, with or without fibrosis, on their liver biopsy. Therapy is easy to justify in ill patients and those at greatest risk of disease progression. It is also most likely to cost-effective in such patients. On the other hand, therapy, which is likely to be long-term, is difficult to justify in patients with mild histologic disease who would have a low risk of disease progression without treatment. This area is controversial. The observation of higher early response to treatment in patients with minimal disease fuels the argument to initial treatment early, but does not address the high cost of treatment in patients who do not usually require any intervention.

Non-response

Approximately half of all patients will not respond to interferon using a standard regimen. Few alternatives exist for these patients. If the patient has not responded after the first 12 weeks of treatment, escalation of the dose to 10 million units will result in response in about 20% of patients. However, this strategy is associated with the high cost and side effects, and should therefore be reserved for those who have aggressive liver disease or incapacitation symptoms. The emerging role of treatment adjuncts is discussed above.

Relapse

Most patients who respond to treatment will relapse. Although initial reports suggest that as many as only half of responders maintained the initial response to interferon, it is now clear that only 20-30% will maintain normal ALT levels for 6-12 months. Additionally, recent data has suggested that virologic relapse occurs even more commonly and many patients who continue to maintain normal ALT levels may actually be viremic and have active liver disease. These disturbing observations reinforce the need for effective identification of relapse with virologic tools and re-treatment to maintain control of infection and active liver disease. Unfortunately, the best way to treat relapse is not clear. Although almost all patients will again normalize their ALT levels when retreated, it is not clear whether repeated 6 month courses, a titrated long-term maintenance regimen, or some other schedule will best serve the patient. Long-term re-treatment with a fixed dose is clearly not well tolerated and is associated with frequent breakthrough (see below). An international multicenter study (US, Canada, France, Spain, Australia) is currently underway to determine the best way to retreat and maintain remission in interferon-responsive patients.

Breakthrough

In reported trials of interferon, between 0-50% of patients have demonstrated a phenomenon known as breakthrough. Breakthrough occurs in patients who normalized their serum ALT levels in the first weeks of treatment but demonstrate re-evaluation of ALT despite ongoing therapy. It is essentially a relapse during treatment. These episodes are usually associated with reappearance of detectable HCV RNA and appear to be emergence of resistance to the effects of Interferon. The cause of this phenomenon is unclear. Naturalizing anti-

Interferon antibodies are responsible for a few cases, particularly with some recombinant Interferon not approved for hepatitis treatment in this country. These cases might also be due to loss of host response to the virus. However, it is likely that most cases result from changes in the virus itself, which render it resistant to the effects of Interferon. This remains to be confirmed.

Definition of Response

The currently accepted definition of response to interferon is normalization of the serum ALT levels at the end of treatment. This definition was arbitrarily defined by investigators in the interferon studies initiated before the identification of the HCV agent. Obviously, documentation of viremia was lacking. The availability of serologic markers of HCV replication (HCV RNA by RT-PCR) confirmed that biochemical response (Normal ALT) was usually associated with a virologic response (negative serum HCV RNA). However, it has recently become apparent that exceptions occur and are associated with early relapse. Additionally, virologic relapse always precedes biochemical relapse, sometimes by months or years. It is clear that the definition of response and relapse needs to be revised to include HCV RNA. Trials are currently underway which will test the appropriateness of various combinations of serologic, biochemical and virologic markers of response, remission, and relapse.

SPECIAL PATIENT GROUPS

Decompensated Cirrhosis

Interferon treatment of decompensated cirrhosis due to hepatitis B is a risky proposition because of the possibility of further decompensation or infection with the flare in ALT, which occurs shortly after beginning treatment. Early experiences with treatment of decompensated cirrhosis due to Hepatitis C indicate that interferon can be administered to most of these patients with good results and no risk of further decompensation (Balart, personal communication). Synthetic function improves in responding patients. Cytopenia and infection may limit therapy in some.

HIV infected patients

HIV co-infected patients have an increased risk of liver failure from chronic Hepatitis C. HCV RNA levels increase over time after HIV seroconversion, particularly once immunodeficiency ensues. HIV and HCV co-infected patients appear to respond no differently to interferon than do patients not infected with HIV, although no study has compared response to HCV RNA levels yet. Thus, Interferon treatment should be considered in HIV co-infected patients before onset of manifestations of immunodeficiency.

Hemophiliacs

Between 60-90% of factor-dependent hemophiliacs have serologic evidence of HCV infection. This occurs because factor concentrates are prepared from plasma pooled from hundreds of individuals who, in many cases, are commercially paid donors. HCV infection is most prevalent in those who have received greater volumes of concentrate, especially of unpasteurized products, and is virtually nonexistent in patients who either have not required factor transfusion of have received exclusively vapor-treated plasma concentrates of recombinant clotting factors. About half of infected patients have abnormal serum ALT levels. Interferon treatment is as effective in this patient population as it is in others and does not appear to be associated with any unique problems. The question of whether or not such patients should have a biopsy before considering treatment is controversial because of the cost and risks of the procedure in these individuals.

Transplant Recipients

HCV infection is common in organ transplant recipients. The true prevalence of infection is considerably underestimated by the tendency for aminotransferase levels to be low to normal and the insensitivity of antibody-based diagnostic tests in immunosuppressed patients. The natural history of HCV infection in transplant recipients is unknown. However, there is a unique syndrome of fibrosing, cholestatic hepatocellular injury similar to that observed in hepatitis B, which occurs in a subset of patients. The role of interferon in treating HCV infection in transplant recipients is not known. Complete response appears to be unusual and there is a small but real risk of acute graft rejection.

Asymptomatic Carriers

Chronic portal or periportal inflammation (CPH or CAH) occurs in 70-100% of anti-HCV and HCV-RNA positive patients with normal ALT levels. In most, the degree of inflammation is mild. Interferon is currently not indicated for these patients for the following reasons: (1) the natural history of the HCV carrier is not known, but is probably comparable to CPH or mild CAH; (2) markers of response to treatment are not available; and (3) most patients are not symptomatic. The possible availability of affordable markers of HCV replication may make treatment based on monitoring the viral response feasible in the future.

Extrahepatic Disease

Mixed cryoglobulinemia, membranous glomerulonephritis, and porphyria cutanea tarda may all be associated with HCV infection. In the case of cryoglobulinemia, the cryoglobulins and the associated disease improve or disappear in about half of treated patients. Patients who do not respond to interferon require treatment with immunosuppressive agents including prednisone, cytoxan, and/or pheresis. HCV-associated porphyria responds to phlebotomy. The effects of interferon are not yet described.

TREATMENT OF ACUTE HEPATITIS C

There is a growing consensus that Interferon treatment of acute Hepatitis C reduces the risk of chronicity. Four randomized controlled trials have all demonstrated a reduction in the proportion of patients with either abnormal ALT levels or detectable HCV RNA following a 4-12 week course of Interferon. Although most "responders" maintain their response, some early responders have evidence of infection at a later follow-up. Unfortunately, such patients are rarely identified since acute infection is usually unapparent and it is impractical to serially screen patients with identifiable risk factors.

FUTURE TREATMENT STRATEGIES

Considerable progress has been made in the therapy of chronic hepatitis C in the few years since the identification of this virus. While interferon treatment is quite effective by antiviral standards, there is no doubt that the currently approved regimen is far from optimal. A great deal of work remains in order to better define the clinical guidelines for the use of interferon in patients with chronic Hepatitis C. It is likely that strategies will develop that individualize treatment regimens according to patient characteristics (body size, histology, etc.) and the predominant viral isolate (genotype and level). Better markers of treatment response will allow fine-tuning of the treatment duration and dose. Ongoing trials will hopefully identify the utility of viral markers of response and determine the optimal way to manage the treatment of the infection over the long- term. Finally, new classes of therapeutic agents such as protease inhibitors, antisense compounds, and therapeutic vaccines will eventually find their way to clinical trials.

REFERENCES

TREATMENT OF CHRONIC HEPATITIS C

Standard Therapy

- Hoofnagle JH, Mullen KD, Jones DB, et al. Treatment of chronic non-A, non-B hepatitis with recombinant human alpha interferon: A preliminary report. New Engl J Med 1986; 315:1575-1578.

- Davis GL, Balart LA, and Schiff ER, et al. Treatment of chronic hepatitis C with recombinant interferon alpha: A multicenter randomized, controlled trial. New Engl J Med 1989; 321:1501-1506.

- Marcellin P, Boyer N, Giostra, et al. Recombinant human alpha- interferon in patients with chronic non A non B hepatitis: a multicenter randomized controlled trial from France. Hepatology 1991; 13:393-397.

- Causse x, Godinot H, Ouzan D, et al. Comparison of 1 or 3 MU of Interferon alfa-2b and placebo in patients with chronic non-A non-B hepatitis. Gastroenterology 1991; 101:497-502.

- TinÅ½ F, Margin S, Craxi A, Pagliaro L. Interferon for non-A, non- B chronic Hepatitis: a meta-analysis of randomized clinical trials. J Hepatol 1991; 13:192-199.

Alternative regimens: Higher dose, Longer duration

- Beloqui O, Prieto J, Suarez M, Gil B, Qian CH, Garcia N, Civeira MP. N-acetyl cysteine enhances the response to interferon-alpha in chronic hepatitis C: a pilot study. J Interferon Res 1993; 13:279-282.

- Kakumu S, Yoshioka K, Wakita T, Ishikawa T, Takayanagi M, Higashi Y. A pilot study of ribavirin and interferon beta for the treatment of chronic hepatitis C. Gastroenterology 1993; 105:507- 512.

- Liaw YF, Sheen IS, Lin SM, Chen TJ, Chu CM. Effects of prednisone pretreatment in Interferon alfa therapy for patients with chronic non-A, non-B (C) hepatitis. Liver 1993; 13:46-50.

Alternatives to Interferon

- Camps J, Garcia N, Riezu-Boj JI, Civiera MP, Prieto J. Ribavirin in the treatment of chronic hepatitis C unresponsive to alfa interferon. J Hepatol 1993; 19:408-412.

- Bodenheimer HC, Lindsay K, Davis GL, et al. Ribavirin treatment of chronic hepatitis C. Hepatology 1994; 20:(abstract in press).

SPECIAL PATIENT GROUPS

Decompensated Cirrhosis

- Dimopoulou M, Fafoutis K, Basiliou K, Ketikoglou J, Karvountzis G. Interferon alfa-2a for decompensated liver disease caused by either chronic hepatitis B or C: preliminary results of a pilot study. Gut 1993; 34 (suppl. 2): S104-105.

HIV infected patients

- Eyster ME, Diamondstone LS, Lien JM, Ehmann WC, Quan S, Goedert JJ. The natural history of hepatitis C virus infection in multitransfused hemophiliacs: Effects of co-infection with human immunodeficiency virus. Acquir Immune Defic Syndr 1993; 6:602.

- Eyster ME, Fried MW, DiBisceglie AM, Goedert JJ. Increasing HCV RNA levels in hemophiliacs: Relationship to HIV infection and liver disease. Blood 1994; (in press).

- Boyer N, Marcellin P. Degott C, Degos F, Saimot AG, Erlinger S, Benhamou JP. Recombinant interferon-alpha for chronic hepatitis C in patients positive for antibody to human immunodeficiency virus. J Infect Dis 1992; 165:723-726.

Hemophiliacs

- Makis M, Preston FR, Triger DR, Underwood JC, Westlake L, Adelman MI. A randomized controlled trial of recombinant interferon-alpha in chronic hepatitis C in hemophiliacs. Blood 1991; 78:1672-1677.

Transplant Recipients

- Lim HL, Lau GK, Davis GL, Dolson DJ, Lau JYN. Cholestatic hepatitis leading to hepatic failure in patients with organ- transmitted hepatitis C virus infection. Gastroenterology 1994; 106:248-251.

- Ferrel LD, Wright TL, Roberts J, Ascher N, Lake J. Hepatitis C viral infection in liver transplant recipients. Hepatology 1992; 16:865-876.

• Wright HI, Gavaler JS, Van Thiel DH. Preliminary experience with alpha-2b interferon therapy of viral hepatitis in liver allograft recipients. Transplantation 1992; 53:121-124.

Asymptomatic Carriers

• Naito M, Hayashi N, Hagiwara H, Hiram N, Kasahara A, Fusamato H, Kamada T. Serum hepatitis C virus RNA quantity and histological features of hepatitis C virus carriers with persistently normal ALT levels. Hepatology 1994; 19:871-875.

Extrahepatic Disease

• Lunel F, Musset L, and Cacoub P, et al. Cryoglobulinemia in chronic liver diseases: role of hepatitis C virus and liver damage. Gastroenterology 1994; 106:1291-1300.

TREATMENT OF ACUTE HEPATITIS C

• Viladomiu L, Genesca J, and Estaban JI, et al. Interferon alpha in acute post transfusion hepatitis C: a randomized controlled trial. Hepatology 1992; 15:767-769.

• Omata M, Yokosuka O, Takano S et al. Resolution of acute hepatitis C after therapy with natural beta interferon. Lancet 1991; 338:914-915.

• Lampertico P, Rumi M, Romeo R, Craxi A, Soffrededini R, Biassoni D, Colombo M. A multicenter randomized controlled trial of recombinant interferon alpha-2b in patients with acute transfusion- associated hepatitis C. Hepatology 1994; 19:19-22.

- Tassopoulos NC, Koutelou MG, Papatheodoridis G, et al. Recombinant human interferon alfa-2b treatment for acute non-A, non-B hepatitis. Gut 1993; 34:S130-132.

Copyright C 1997 The American Liver Foundation

Appendix B

HEPASTAT™

Recent scientific studies on the milk thistle have verified traditional Chinese and European herbalists' use of this plant for its beneficial effect on the liver. We have combined this herb with seven others to give you a formula designed to nutritionally support you system. Only high quality herbs, which pass our rigid standards, are used. HEPASTAT™ does not contain any artificial ingredients. In order to satisfy our many different customers and their nomenclature requests we have listed the herbs: scientific name/common name/Chinese herb name. Listed below are the herbs and the traditional indications of the same.

Scientific Name	*Common Name*	*Chinese Name*
Bupleurum Chinese DC	*Bupleurum*	*Chai-hu*
Scutellaria baicalensis Georgi	*Scute*	*Huang-chin*
Paeonia lactiflora Pall	*White peony root*	*Chih-shao*
Isatis indigotica Fort	*Isatidis*	*Ta-ching-yeh*
Astragalus membranaceus	*Astragalus*	*Huang-chi*
Silybum marianum Gaertn	*Milk thistle*	*Shui-fei-ji*
Apis mellifera L.	*Royal jelly*	*Fon-hwan-chiang*
Glycyrrhiza glabra L.	*Licorice*	*Gan-cao*

Bupleurum Chinese DC—"anti-pyretic; liver qi (energy) stagnation; collapse of spleen qi (energy)"

Scutellaria baicalensis Georgi—"removes toxins; gastroenteritis; water retention"

Paeonia lactiflora Pall—"anti-bacterial; anti-spasmodic; anti-inflammatory; analgesic; tranquilizing; lowers blood pressure"

Isatis indigotica Fort—"cools blood; removes toxins; cleanses and soothes throat"

Astragalus membranaceus—"increases production of white blood cells; strengthens immune response; anti-bacterial; energy tonic"

Silybum marianum Gaertn—"protects intact liver cells or cells not yet irreversibly damaged"

Apis mellifera L.—"phlegm expectorant; abscess emollient; ulcer detergent; helps relieve arthritis pain"

Glycyrrhiza glabra L.—"anti-inflammatory for arthritic or allergic conditions; digestive stimulant; lung disorders"

THE POWER OF HERBS

For thousands of years, ancient cultures have used the power of herbs to support the functions of the body. Much of the continuing work done by modern research substantiates the wisdom of the ancients in their application and use of herbs. Single herbs used alone often will not have the same effect as when combined in a formula; a synergy is created. To achieve this synergy was a measure of the ancient herbalists' ability. Successful formulas often were closely held and passed on to the next generation. Modern science is just beginning to unlock the ancients' wisdom.

HEPASTAT™

This herbal formula is designed to reduce liver damage and help recovery form infection caused by toxic agents such as: HAV, HBV, HCV, HDV, and HEV. Its mechanisms of action include immune regulation and enhancing the body's own ability to protect the liver.

Its pharmacological actions are summarized below:

1. Enhances immune function, activates macrophage activity, induces interferon and Interleuken-3 production.

2. Destroys hepatitis virus (inside infected liver cells) and inhibits viral reproduction.

3. Improves hepatic cell membrane function and decreases hepatic cell damage by reducing membrane permeability.

4. Enhances glycogen synthesis.

5. Improves microcirculation and stimulates bile secretion.

6. Improves appetite and GI functions.

Special notes: (1) it is effective for prevention prior to exposure to hepatic virus. (2) Not suitable for hepatoma patients.

Milk Thistle (silybum marianum) is used in Europe in both over-the-counter and prescription medications to treat a variety of liver ailments. According to medical literature published overseas the herb, known scientifically as silymarin, has been used successfully in treating hepatitis and reversing liver damage caused by cirrhosis, drugs and toxins (without side effects).

The herb has conclusively been shown to be liver protective and regenerative even against one of the most virulent liver toxins known, the death cap mushroom (amanita phalloides). In its early stages of growth, this mushroom resembles the common agaricus and may be mistakenly eaten. The result is usually fatal. Pretreatment of animals with silymarin gives 100% protection against this poison. Milt thistle is also effective against chronic liver cirrhosis, necroses and hepatitis. It is hypolipidemic and lowers fat deposits in the liver of animals (9).

Hepata*Trope has been used successfully in the treatment of cholesterol levels. To assist the liver in cholesterol lowering, case studies have shown when taking Hepata*Trope along with Phytosterol Complex, the level of cholesterol has dropped as much as 50 points a month.

The largest of the internal organs, the liver, "weighs in" at 2.5 to 3 pounds. It is suspended behind the ribs on the upper right side of the abdomen and spans almost the entire width of the body.

Hepata*Trope™

Lipotropic Formula

Product No. SC108 Size: 90 capsules

NDC51821-979-90

Each Capsule Contains:

*Milk Thistle (Silybum marianum)...100mg.
*Choline Bitartrate.....150mg.
*Inositol.....75mg.
Vitamin B-6.....5mg.
Vitamin B-12.....200mcg.
Folic Acid.....200mcg.
Pantothenic Acid.....125mg.
PABA.....50mg.
Vitamin C.....50 mg.
*DI-Methionine.....50mg.
*Betaine3HCI.....60mg.
*Black Radish.....50mg.
*Green Beet Leaf Powder.....30mg.
*Chionanthus.....30mg.
*Magnesium Aspartate.....25mg.
*Celandine (Shelidonium majas).....15mg.

Suggested Usage: For Adults, 1 or 2 capsules, three times daily or as directed by your licensed Practitioner.

Lipotropics Prevent Fat accumulation in the Liver

The liver removes fatty acids from diet or from deposits by degrading and oxidizing them when the body must call on fat as a major energy source. Lipotropic factors such as those found in Hepata*Trope must be active to prevent abnormal accumulation of fats in the liver. By a process of transmethylation, these lipotropic agents promote the production of lipoproteins, which transfer the fatty acids out of the liver (2).

Normal liver fat is 5% to 15%, whereas, a diabetic's liver is 25% to 35% fat. The percentage of liver fat may also be increased by:

- Excessive Alcohol Consumption
- Birth Control Pills
- Estrogen Usage
- High Vitamin B-1 and B-12 Intake
- Colbalt Treatments

Conditions that can result from liver dysfunction include:

- Menstrual irregularities
- Constipation
- Hypertension
- Blood sugar metabolic imbalance
- Fatigue
- Glaucoma
- Arteriosclerosis
- Hepatitis
- Jaundice

Hormone conjugation also occurs in the liver. By keeping the liver healthy, **Hepata*Trope** aids in this reaction. Estrogen can be carcinogenic if it is not conjugated. Calcium, protein, mineral, and fat metabolism are all regulated by components of conjugated estrogen. An unhealthy, fatty or cirrhotic liver cannot perform these functions efficiently.

Hepata*Trope is Targeted to Lipid Metabolism and Liver Function

In addition to the protective and regenerative Mild Thistle herb, Scientific Bio-Logics has included in the **Hepata*Trope** formula specific vitamins, minerals, amino acids and herbs, each of which is targeted to lipid metabolism and healthy liver function. These nutrients aid the liver and gall bladder in metabolism of lipids and conjugation of hormones such as estradiol. **Choline**, considered one of the B vitamins, functions with inositol as a basic constituent of lecithin. It appears to be associated primarily with utilization of fats and cholesterol in the body. It prevents fats from accumulating in the liver and facilitates the movement of fats into the cells. Choline combines with fatty acids and phosphoric acid within the liver to form lecithin. It improves liver and gallbladder function and helps prevent gallstones (3). **Inositol**, like choline, is a constituent of lecithin, which is needed to move fats from the liver to the cells. High intake of caffeine may create an inositol shortage in the body (3). **Vitamin B-6**, is involved in the metabolism of fats and fatty acids, especially the essential unsaturated fatty acids. Birth control pills increase the risk of gallstones, which can be caused by oxalic acid toxicity. Vitamin B-6 detoxifies oxalic acid

(7). **Vitamin B-12** and **Folic Acid** are used in the synthesis of methionine and choline. The coenzyme of vitamin B-12 is a carrier of methyl groups and hydrogen and is necessary for carbohydrate, protein and fat metabolism. Because of its methyl transfer role, vitamin B-12 is active in the synthesis of the amino acid methionine from its precursor, homocysteine. The coenzyme transfers methyl groups from methyl folate; a derivative of folic acid, to homeocystine and methionine is formed. Because methionine is needed in choline synthesis, B-12 plays a secondary role in the lipid pathway. A choline deficiency that causes fatty liver can be prevented by vitamin B-12 and the other methyl donors – betaine, methionine folic aced (3). **PABA**, para-aminobenzoic acid, stimulates the intestinal bacteria, enabling them to produce folic acid, which in turn aids in the production of pantothenic acid (3). **Pantothenic Acid** has clinical application in lipogenesis formation of cholesterol, formation of steroid hormones and detoxification of drugs (2). **Magnesium** is necessary for coenzyme A reaction. The mineral has shown to enhance enzymatic activity in the liver (4). Vitamin and trace mineral deficiencies lower coenzyme activity (1). Magnesium in case studies has been credited with dissolving gallstones (7). Alcohol consumption increases the dietary need for magnesium threefold (4). **Celandine** is primarily used as a liver-detoxifying herb for the treatment of hepatitis, jaundice, cancer, psoriasis, eczema and skin problems (9). **Chionanthus** is a mild stimulant for the bowels and a tonic that strengthens or invigorates organs or the entire organism. This herb has a beneficial effect on the kidneys and liver, including acute and chromic liver inflammation and cirrhosis of the liver (6). It has been used successfully in treating menstrual disorders, hepatic derangements, jaundice, enlarged spleen and jaundice with arrest of menses (5). **Black Radish** appears to help speed up the flow of bile and has a detoxifying effect of the liver and spleen (7). **Beet Leaves** have been found to increase bile flow as well as to aid in carbohydrate and fat metabolism (7). **Betaine** is a source of methyl groups. It is used in the liver for the detoxification of free radicals and other reactive by-products (7). **Methionine** acts as a methyl donor and antioxidant in liver tissues and aids healing and detoxification of these tissues (7). Its' primary lipotropic function is to prevent excess fat accumulations in the liver by increasing lecithin production (8).

No specific claim is made for this nutritional preparation. Any recommendations for its use are based solely upon the discretion of the doctor. The information contained within is based upon authoritative and reliable source. As such, disagreement is possible.

REFERENCES

1. Blackwoods Materia Medica, Economic Homceo Pharmacy (1959).
2. Williams, Sue Rodwell, Nutrition and Diet Therapy, C.W. Mosby Co. (1969).
3. Nutrition Search, Inc., Nutrition Almanac, McGraw Hill (1975).

4. Heinz International Research Center, Heinz Nutritional Data, Heinz 1972.

5. Colimore, Benjamin and Sarah Stewart, Nutrition and Your Body, Light Wave (1974).

6. Clark, Linda, Handbook of Natural Remedies for Common Ailments, Devia Adair (1976).

7. Boericke, William, Pocket Manual of Homeopathic Materia Medica, Boericke & Runyon (1972).

8. Garrison, Robert H, jr. and Somer, Elizabeth, The Nutrition Desk Reference Keats Publishing, New Canaan, CT, 1985.

9. Tierra, Michael, The Way of Herbs, Pocket Books, New York, NY 1990

Appendix C

Citation: Business Wire, Nov. 18, 1994 p11180037

Title: Significant results in hepatitis C study with thymosin alpha 1 and interferon alpha combination therapy.

Subjects: Pharmaceutical industry Product development

Thymosin Testing

Hepatitis C Drug therapy

Companies: SciClone Pharmaceuticals Inc. Product development

Reference #: A15878838

Full Test COPYRIGHT Business Wire 1994

SAN MATEO, Calif.-(Business Wire)-Nov. 18, 1994-SciClone Pharmaceuticals Inc.

(NASDAQ:SCLN) Friday commented on results from a randomized, placebo-controlled, double blind phase III study in chronic hepatitis C patients receiving a combination therapy of thymosin alpha 1 and interferon alpha-2B.

A life-table analysis showed almost 50% of the 65 patients had complete normalization of ALT in the thymosin combination treated group and in less than 20% of the interferon-only treated group.

The data described studies performed at the Fitzsimons Army Medical Center, Aurora, Colo., and the Walter Reed Medical Center, Washington D.C., and was presented by Dr. Kenneth Sherman and colleagues at the 45th Annual Meeting of the American Association for the Study of Liver Diseases (AASLD) held in Chicago this week.

"We observed a statistically significant reduction in ALT levels in the combination group and significant complete normalization of ALT levels, as compared to the interferon only and placebo groups, " said Dr. Sherman, currently an associate professor at the University of Cincinnati Medical Center. "We also observed significant early virologic response in patients treated with combination therapy when compared to the interferon arm."

The complete normalization of ALT levels observed in the combination treatment group is a key observation in the trial since the approval of interferon, the only drug approved by the Food and Drug Administration (FDA) to treat hepatitis C was based on this primary endpoint of normalized ALT levels.

The on-going study involved three arms: combination therapy with thymosin and interferon, interferon alone, and a placebo control group. At the end of the six-month treatment phase, the combination treatment group also demonstrated statistical significance in the loss of hepatitis C RNA virus and improvement in histology when compared to placebo.

The data reported this week is in accord with data from a separate, previously reported study by Dr. Guido Rasi of the University Tor Vergata in Rome. The 15-patient, open label Italian study used combination therapy with thymosin alpha 1 and alpha interferon to treat chronic hepatitis C patients. The data from this study showed reduction in ALT and RNA levels and improvement in histology.

SciClone Pharmaceuticals Inc. is developing thymosin alpha 1 under the trade name ZADAXIN. The company has clinical development, manufacturing and marketing rights for ZADAXIN. SciClone is engaged in the acquisition and development of pharmaceuticals to market in targeted countries worldwide.

The company's primary focus is on the development of therapeutics for infectious diseases including hepatitis B and C, cancers and immune system disorders that are life threatening and place major cost burdens on the world healthcare systems.

CONTACT: SciClone Pharmaceuticals Inc., San Mateo
Michelle E. Slade, 415/358-3456

Appendix D

Alfalfa Leaf Ingredients

Vitamins:	**Minerals:**	**Amino Acids**
Beta Carotene	Chromium	Arginine
Vitamin B-1	Calcium	Alanine
Vitamin B-2	Copper	Aspartic Acid
Niacin	Iodine	Cysteine
Vitamin B-6	Iron	Glutamic
Vitamin B-12	Magnesium	Acid
Pantothenic	AcidManganese	Glycine
Folic Acid	Molybdenum	Histidine
Biotin	Phosphorus	*Isoleucine
P.A.B.A.	Potassium	*Leucine
Inositol	Selenium	*Lysine
Choline*	Sodium	*Methionine
Vitamin C	Zinc	Phenylalanine
Vitamin E		Proline
Vitamin		Serine
(Phylloquinone)		*Threonine
		Tyrosine
		*Valine

*Denotes an essential amino acid

Pigments:
Chlorophyll
Xanthophyll

Addendum 1

By Jackie Judd

ABCNEWS.com

Sept. 17, 1999_____Multiple sclerosis and central nervous disorders can lead to paralysis, slurred speech and vision problems. While there's no cure, researchers at the Mayo Clinic have developed a treatment that may help people with the most severe cases.

A handful of people, like MS patient Andrew Grant, have already seen the benefits of the new treatment. Though he was completely immobile two years ago, Grant is up and moving again thanks to an experimental approach called plasma exchange.

He and 18 other patients with severely damaged nervous systems had blood removed. A special machine then separated the cells from the plasma, or liquid part of the blood. Plasma from healthy donors was purified until it contained just one protein called albumin. The donor plasma and the original cells were mixed together and put back into the patients.

This exchange was repeated seven times over a two-week period. For this group of severely disabled patients, standard anti-inflammatory treatment hadn't helped. But plasma exchange allowed many of them to regain their speech, as well as movement in their arms and legs.

"We had a robust, major effect in 40 percent of the patients," says Dr. Brian Weinshenker, a Mayo Clinic neurologist and the study's lead researcher.

In those who were helped, the effect was almost immediate.

On day 14, Grant could get out of bed and walk with assistance. Six months later, he could walk on his own. When he felt his foot move, he says, "I put a big old smile on my face."

Doctors are not entirely sure why this treatment succeeded. An early theory is the patients' plasma contained harmful antibodies that allowed the disease to progress at a rapid pace. The replacement plasma stopped that process.

"I think it's just dramatic," says Weinshenker, "how touching the plasma alone, without doing anything to the cells, can affect an immediate recovery from a neurological disability."

He and his colleagues presented the results of their study, which was funded by the National Institute of Health, at a medical conference today in Basel, Switzerland. They'll publish their findings in the December issue of Annals of Neurology.

The researchers are careful to point out, however, that the new treatment isn't for everyone with MS, and it's not a cure. "Plasma exchange should be considered only for those patients who have severe, acute attacks of MS that are not responsive to high-dose steroid treatments," Weinshenker says.

Addendum 2

By John McKenzie

ABCNEWS.com

February 28, 2000_____It usually begins in medical school. Students receive drug company pens, and clocks, and coffee mugs.

When they become doctors, the gifts they receive often increase in value. Drug samples; tickets to ball games; dinners for doctors and their families, even all-expense-paid trips to ski or beach resorts to "consult" with drug company representatives are being given out.

"The companies and sales reps will tell you, " says Dr. Seth Landefeld of the University of California, San Francisco, "you deserve to go out to a particularly nice place, to a nice conference."

It is all part of an intense marketing effort. Each drug company tries to convince doctors of the benefits of its medications, so the doctors, in turn, might prescribe them to you.

By one published estimate, drug companies last year spent an average of $13,000 on every physician in the country, which adds up to more than $8 billion. Drug companies now employ 70,000 sales representatives, which means one sales representative for every nine doctors.

"It is important for pharmaceutical company representatives to be able to help educate doctors about the medicines that the company that discovers and develops them, know best," says Judy Bello, a pharmaceutical industry representative.

The Question is: Do the gifts and entertainment that drug companies offer lead some doctors to practice bad medicine?

"It's the gifts, it's the influence that's the problem," explains Dr. Robert Tenery of the American Medical Association. "It's creating incentives that may change the way doctors practice medicine and why they prescribe certain medications."

And, potentially, at the patient's expense.

A recent analysis by the Journal of the American Medical Association of 16 different studies showed that doctors courted by drug companies were more likely to engage in "non-rational" prescribing. In other words, they were more likely to order a drug that was more expensive, or less effective, than what the patient actually needed. The doctors were also more likely -- in some cases, 20 times more likely -- to ask a hospital to add the company's drug to the hospital inventory -- even though most of the requested drugs "presented little or no therapeutic advantage."

Still, most doctors deny that they are influenced by gifts.

"This is a very hot-button issue," says Landefeld. "There are few buttons in medicine you could push that gets doctors stirred up faster."

In part, because many doctors suggest they're too clever to be manipulated by a pharmaceutical company.

"I've worked in places where we've had policies saying we will accept gifts but we won't be influenced by them," says Dr. Allen Shaughnessy of the Medical College of Pennsylvania. "And I try to point out that that's impossible. The two go hand in hand."

The American Medical Association, the country's largest doctor's group, tried to address this problem several years ago. Together with the pharmaceutical industry, the AMA put out guidelines that say gifts to doctors should serve a genuine "educational function" and not be of "substantial" value, usually defined as more than $100.

But these guidelines are voluntary, and the AMA now concedes that many "troubling practices" returned.

Triumph Over Hepatitis C
A Non-Profit Organization

For Information Regarding Tax Deductible Contributions
Or for Product Sales and Ordering
contact Lloyd Wright:

Email: lloydhepcfree@msn.com
Website: www.hepatitiscfree.com
Toll Free 877-676-1615

As a courtesy to my readers, I am happy to provide everything in my remedy at wholesale prices. This is done for your convenience as I had a very difficult time finding many of the items and was charged outrageous prices for others.

Thank You for your support!